T0333047

Your Mental Health

Your Mental Health

Understanding Depression,
Anxiety, PTSD, Eating Disorders
and Self-Destructive Behaviour

Edited by Tony Westbrook and Chris Brady

Vermilion
LONDON

Published in 2023 by Vermilion, an imprint of Ebury Publishing
20 Vauxhall Bridge Road,
London SW1V 2SA

Vermilion is part of the Penguin Random House group of companies
whose addresses can be found at global.penguinrandomhouse.com

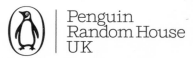

Penguin
Random House
UK

Text © Enigma Holdings Group Limited

Chris Brady and Tony Westbrook have asserted their rights to be
identified as the authors of the work in accordance with the Copyright,
Designs and Patents Act 1988
Lead writer: Franca Davenport

This edition first published by Vermilion in 2023

www.penguin.co.uk

A CIP catalogue record for this book is available from the British Library

ISBN 9781785044656

Typeset in 10/14.5pt DIN 2014 by Jouve (UK), Milton Keynes
Printed and bound in Great Britain by Clays Ltd, Elcograf S.p.A.

The authorised representative in the EEA is Penguin Random House Ireland,
Morrison Chambers, 32 Nassau Street, Dublin D02 YH68

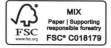

Penguin Random House is committed to a
sustainable future for our business, our readers
and our planet. This book is made from Forest
Stewardship® certified paper.

contents

foreword

BY TONY WESTBROOK

I've been a doctor now for some 30 years but I still remember my medical student days at Mapperley Psychiatric Hospital in Nottingham. Things have changed a lot since then. In the past, long-stay patients at these institutions were subjected to lobotomies and other treatments that would now seem barbaric. These people were permanently damaged as a result and were consequently never going to get better. It's so different to my current role as a Consultant Orthopaedic Surgeon, where I provide curative treatments for many joint problems, such as fractures or arthritis, to reduce pain, increase function and allow people to return to normal activities. I see my job as enhancing and not hindering quality of life.

The majority of those admitted to mental health institutions such as Mapperley were long-stay patients, essentially being kept out of sight of society. They had chronic conditions such as manic depression or schizophrenia. Just being a bit depressed wouldn't get you accepted; you had to be either suicidal or close to it. But at that time there was a serious lack of understanding of the different mental health issues we now know about and discuss. We didn't talk about eating disorders or even PTSD in the 1970s and 1980s. Sufferers must have come out of two world wars, horribly scarred by their experiences, and simply ordered to get on with life. Why? Because it didn't yet exist as a condition. This is why researching mental health issues and deepening our understanding is so important. If we do not, there's no telling how many people in need of support are being failed.

There is nothing more mysterious than the human brain, in everything it does and how it functions. Mental health is obviously very much bound up in that, but there is still much that we don't yet fully understand. Why does one family member suffer with anxiety, depression, or an eating disorder for no obvious reason, when the others are little affected by poor mental health. Some may say it's just in their nature, or their make-up. But why, when a family group has shared genes, do some struggle more than others? These are answers we will only be able to answer with research and inquiry.

How do we explain the coping mechanisms and resilience of certain individuals that prevents them from transcending into poor mental health? In 2017 I was part of the team that treated Billy Monger, a young racing driver who had a horrific accident at Donington Park Race Track, which resulted in both his legs being amputated. If anyone demonstrates the power of positivity and making the most of every day, it is Billy. Speaking on the *Power of Positivity* podcast, he said: 'the way I look at my accident in general is that this is life, one of those things. The injuries were visually quite shocking but I have to bounce back. I don't like to look back on things, I like to look forward to the future. I see it as that was meant to be.'[1]

This is an incredible way of dealing with things. The reframing of an event. I don't really understand why Billy has coped so well, inspiring others along the way like he has without the significant psychological trauma one might expect. But as we have learned from other aspects of mental health, it is only through further research that we will achieve true understanding.

When I look back on my attachment on the psychiatric wards, I remember dreary environments, but the writer Bill Bryson, who worked at Holloway Sanatorium in 1970s, had very different memories. In his book *Notes From a Small Island*, he described the hospital as 'the most perfect thing I'd ever seen. It was the best, it was just such a brilliant, enlightened way of treating people, who couldn't cope in society, and they were comfortably housed and institutionalized. It was a beautiful place that had beautiful gardens that were maintained by the patients and, insofar as they could, they had quite fulfilling lives, obviously within the confinement that they were experiencing.'[2]

While it seemed at the time that patients were having a good experience, the way mental health issues were treated was very different and understanding was simply not there. Thankfully we are now at a stage where patients admitted for mental health reasons are generally expected to make a full recovery and reintegrate back into society.

There is much that I feel the medical profession can do to improve the way we care for any patient, irrespective of whether they are physically or psychologically unwell. Every hospital, not just in Britain but in the world, needs brightening up. That alone will make things better for staff and patients. Giving people a comfortable and comforting environment is important and tends to be overlooked. Current paediatric wards are a great example of best practice. They incorporate the wiring and tubes and everything that says 'hospital' into murals painted on the wall. While adults may not necessarily need Mickey Mouse painted on a wall in their ward, a lot more can be done to give patients a supportive environment where they are given the best chance of recovery.

I hope that, in time, we will continue to deepen our understanding on mental health, an area where there is still much more to learn. In 50 years from now people may well look back on our current practices and find them just as barbaric as we do those of the 1970s. Trying to develop greater levels of understanding about mental health is precisely why this book was written. Trying to eliminate the noise in order to concentrate on the signals is an awesome task, but one worth the effort.

We know an understanding of mental health can be particularly difficult as medicine is an imperfect science. The surgeon and writer Atul Gawande, author of *Complications* and *The Checklist Manifesto* comments on this. He says: 'We seek to know, understand and comprehend every facet of the human body, but the simple fact is, we don't and perhaps can't. It simply isn't the case that if you add all the right ingredients or component parts, and if you create the right environments, you will be guaranteed the product you want. Some elements of medicine are more predictable than others, in some the outcome can be more reliably influenced, but nowhere is there more uncertainty, or more haziness than in the realms of mental health.'[3]

This reinforces my opinion that we need to research more to gain a greater understanding. I hope that by reading this book, you will start to develop a greater insight into your own mental health.

preface

BY PETER GEORGE AND
ANDY LEAVER

Our role in this book has been to gather together those people
we believe could deliver a product that would enable greater
understanding of the mental health issues that currently bedevil
us. Why we wanted to do so is quite complex and multifaceted.
As a biochemist, Peter has always been intrigued by what
physiological aspects drive good or bad mental health. Being
involved in the pharmaceutical industry, we wondered whether
the various issues were 'curable' or at least 'treatable' through
pharmaceutical intervention and, if so, what modes of action that
would involve. As an employer we were fascinated by the biases
inflicted upon those of difference, be it colour, race, sex, religion,
disability or mental health. Probably what intrigued us most was
whether embracing or ignoring these differences affected the
positive or negative responses of workforces in general – but, to
be honest, ours in particular.

Our first example of this was when Peter met a 12-time
Paralympic gold medallist at a dinner at the Welsh Assembly. He
and an able-bodied Olympian (no medals at this point) were
friends and were writing to Welsh companies looking for
sponsorship. The Paralympian with 12 gold medals had had no
replies and zero success; the as yet un-medalled able-bodied
Olympian had had replies from all and positive responses from
many (he did later win a bronze medal). This seemed unfair.
Sitting to Peter's right was the gold medallist's then-girlfriend,
now wife, who was also disabled. She had qualified as a lawyer

in Scandinavia and had recently qualified in law in the UK, she spoke three languages fluently, but the only job she could secure was working on the checkouts at Tesco. Again, this seemed unfair; they were adamant that people couldn't see beyond their disabilities. That evening Peter agreed to sponsor the athlete and offered a job to his partner. They both ended up working with Peter for many years, have remained firm friends, and she was one of the best employees we ever had.

At the same time, in the company, two people in the same department were requesting leave on health grounds. One was pregnant. For her we had procedures to follow, guidelines to adhere to, and we pulled out all the stops. Everyone was aware of her pregnancy, everyone was supportive and communicative. She was clear that her job would be held for her and that upon her return she could decide what she wanted to do. The other employee had financial and family issues that had led to severe acute mental health issues. The difference in the way this person was treated was embarrassing. No one wanted to talk to them, little support was offered, the manager and HR department were considering dismissing them, there was no offer of time off and the job being kept open.

Once again it seemed unfair. Peter is disappointed to say that at that point he didn't do anything to change things, he just remembers it vividly as something in which he should have intervened. Why don't we treat mental health in the workplace with the same compassion as we use for pregnancy? If we did it would lead to loyal employees who felt valued and supported; it's a missed opportunity. In our subsequent companies, this is something we have addressed, and it has had hugely positive results.

Shortly after this Peter was hit with a family issue. He was busy floating our company on the stock market when his daughter returned from university, clearly unwell. She had left for university a bright, energetic, enthusiastic girl, heading to study International Business Studies. She returned nine months later broken, insular and severely anorexic. It became clear to us over the next two or three years that mental health treatments are inadequate, there is no continuity of care if you move region and standards vary significantly. To this day she has received no acceptable, readily available support or treatment.

Our involvement since with Sporting Force, a charity that supports mental health challenges in ex-military personnel, has confirmed the same. Many have told us that their biggest issue was a lack of continuity of care. Every time they meet with a new healthcare professional, they have to retell their story, and it's like torture, reliving the hell every time. They complain that the standards of care are inadequate and there seems to be no agreement on what type of care is best. And with our involvement with sportspeople who suffer with mental health issues, we've heard the same stories.

But these are just experiences we have had where our life has touched the world of mental health; it doesn't answer the question, 'What drove you to commission this book on standards of care in mental wellbeing?' The answer, as we've said, is complex and multifaceted. It is ALL of the above that sensitised us to the issue; but it is particularly, and not surprisingly, Peter's daughter's pain. What made us think we could or should do something about it, however, was a statistic.

A statistic had changed our lives once before. We had read that 85 per cent of the world's population cannot get access to the medicine they require to treat their disease. We didn't believe this, but on investigation we found it to be true. Most medicines are not licensed in most countries, they are licensed where most commercial sales can be made. Therefore it is true: 85 per cent of people don't get access to the best drugs. This led us to set up our company, Clinigen, which had as its goal to 'Give access to the right medicine, to the right patient at the right time'. Delivering medicines to over 200 countries worldwide led to Clinigen becoming the fastest-growing pharmaceutical company in the UK.

So, when Peter saw a statistic that suggested that 99 per cent of mental health issues are situational, although at first he didn't believe it he looked deeper. It is certainly true that bipolar or psychotic disorders are very rare compared to mood, anxiety or stress disorders, the latter being predominantly situational. In other words, if you improve the situation you can treat the disorder. Suddenly an insurmountable problem seemed surmountable – maybe we could do something about it; maybe we could make a difference. But where to start? The scientist in Peter wanted to go back to root cause analysis. Understand the problem, identify the best ways to treat the problem and then build a system around the facts. This worked in medicine, where standards of care clearly laid out the best path of treatment. It worked in the world of pharmaceuticals and clinical trials, where clear standards led to successful outcomes. In both cases, it worked particularly well if these standards were audited. So, we thought, why couldn't it work here? Step one surely was to have clear standards of care for the vast majority of mental health issues, that 99 per cent!

So here we are. This book is a first step in increasing understanding of the problem. A first step in trying to engage the attention of the research community in an attempt to improve the standards of mental health care, to move the narrative up a level. We don't expect it to stop here. We hope the book will help drive continuous improvement; we hope it manages to change opinions for the better; but most of all we hope it improves someone's life.

introduction

'I have been a stalwart champion of raising mental health awareness for more than 30 years. I never expected to say that there has been a negative impact, which is awareness without real understanding. The purpose of awareness campaigns is to remove the stigma of mental illness and ensure that those suffering get optimum support, as soon as possible. It seems we have reduced the taboo around needing therapy, which is a huge positive, but, in the process, we have opened the floodgates of emotional expression without accurate knowledge of mental health.'

JULIA SAMUEL, THE TIMES, 16 JANUARY 2023

'We're on the cusp of understanding how psychological, social and biological factors interact to put people on different paths towards mental health or mental illness. And that's a very important problem to untangle.'

PROFESSOR ED BULLMORE

HISTORY

It is the aim of this book to increase understanding without affecting the greater awareness that has developed over recent years.

The diagnosis and treatment of mental health conditions is not a new phenomenon, although the names may have changed, from hysteria, shell shock, psychosis, and even demonic possession to the disorders we focus on in this book – depression, anxiety, PTSD, eating disorders and self-destructive behaviours. The treatments have also changed from exorcisms, starvation, dehydrations and various snake oil drugs and medications that are no longer acceptable.

As the centuries passed, isolation from society became popular as a way of removing the patients from sight by placing them in 'insane asylums'. Other versions of mental health treatments included Freudian therapeutic techniques, electroconvulsive therapy (ECT) shock treatment and the dreaded lobotomy and other forms of psychosurgery. Lobotomies are now banned in most countries but were legal in Scandinavia until the 1980s, and the last legal lobotomy in the USA was performed as late as 1967.

Drugs, including whole families of drugs aimed at specific disorders, also gained prominence more recently. The 1970s saw the rise of a drug dependency culture. The benzo (benzodiazepine) family, for example, was primarily targeted at anxiety and became hugely popular and a huge moneymaker for Big Pharma. The benzo family includes such well-known trade names as Librium, Valium and Xanax. Accessing funding to train as a therapist became harder and the proliferation of talking therapies didn't keep up with the widespread use of medication. As the mental health campaigner Dr Heather Ashton has observed, listening to patients became a lost art.

One result of this search for a pharmaceutical magic bullet for mental illness was that drugs that were designed to be taken as short-term (30-day) remedies for difficult times were being repeatedly prescribed for use over decades. In the UK in 2021, antidepressants (predominantly selective serotonin reuptake inhibitors, or SSRIs) were prescribed for close to 10 million people, an increase of 5 per cent over the previous year. The routine response, in particular from under-pressure GPs, became to prescribe a combination of a short course of CBT and antidepressant drugs for everyone experiencing depression. However over 30 per cent of people with depression still report no benefit from current approaches, even if they have tried at least two. This condition is known as treatment-resistant depression.

In the 1940s, grandiose claims were made for psychedelic drugs when Albert Hofmann first proposed that they could be beneficial in the treatment of mental disorders, but enthusiasm quickly waned. Recently, however, there has been a resurgence of interest in the use of these drugs and trials have been showing positive results.

The modern patient now has a full range of 'interventions' from which to choose – from the standard talking therapies and medicines, to nutritional remedies, to 'kindness lessons', social prescribing or the rituals of most of the world's religions. These rituals, which emphasise the value of community and social connection, are bastions against loneliness, a triggering factor for depression. Recent research has found that activities such as attending a place of worship increased resilience, which in turn lowered the risk of symptoms of depression and anxiety. Of course, it is not argued that belief in a God produced these benefits but that the effects of church-going or attending team sports or even playing in a team is the key factor. Indeed, as with many current interventions that have been shown to work, there is still much to be learnt about how they actually take effect.

The many permutations for managing mental health reflect its complexity and the fact that because there is not one single cause it is impossible to have one single magic bullet.

WHY NOW?

Today in the UK, one in four people are impacted by mental illness. This mental health crisis has a debilitating impact on individuals, on families, on communities and on businesses.

A report by the LSE and the Mental Health Foundation has estimated that mental health problems cost the UK economy nearly £120 billion a year, mainly in lost productivity and work absences.[1]

Mental health issues account for the highest amount of time lost through disability globally from all medical causes (26 per cent). Almost the same as the next two highest, musculoskeletal diseases (14 per cent) and neurological and sense-organ conditions (13 per cent), put together.

Close to 75 per cent of mental disorders start before adulthood, but it can take up to 10 years just to get an accurate diagnosis. Twelve per cent of those in conflict situations (domestic, military, first responders) suffer from moderate to severe mental issues. Suicide is the second-highest cause of death in 15–30-year-olds, behind only 'unintentional injuries'. This adds up to 90 deaths per hour or 703,000 suicides per year. Commonly known addictions such as to alcohol and drugs, a significant obstacle to wellbeing, have more recently been joined by the formal recognition of others like gambling, social media, gaming . . . and so it goes on.

However, despite this enormous burden of disease, significantly less has been historically spent on research into understanding and developing effective interventions for mental health disorders. A 2017 report from MQ Mental Health Research found that over 25 times more was spent on cancer research than is spent on ALL mental health research.[2]

Such numbers pose huge challenges for individuals, the workplace and the economic growth every country seeks. However, there is a perception, which may be very close to the reality, that there is a gap between policymakers' well-meaning commitments to improving the nation's mental wellbeing and the real initiatives necessary to tackle the underlying causes of real distress. Investment is needed, not the hand-wringing and verbal sticking plasters that achieve little.

Generally, it is accepted that a lot has changed in the last 10 years – lessons have been learnt that have seen mental health issues become a lot less stigmatised both in practice and in the media. The Covid-19 pandemic may have opened a schism in society when it comes to our mental health, but it did result in an acceleration of collaborative approaches to research and the development of new technology-driven interventions.

All of which helped to drive the commissioning of this book and its purpose. A characteristics-based definition of a 'quiet crisis' is one in which participants are caught unawares by a high threat and have a lack of time to avoid catastrophe. However, all of these characteristics demand that the person/organisation involved *perceives* the threat. It seems that the very term, 'quiet', suggests that mental health is not in crisis because it is not perceived as an imminent threat. If it were, there would be a louder reaction.

PURPOSE

The purpose of this book is not, therefore, to produce a self-help tome – enough of those exist already. The purpose is to enable greater understanding of the issues surrounding the 'quiet crisis'. To demystify, simplify and clarify the extreme complexity of the issues with which human beings must contend. And the numbers do suggest that at some stage of our lives we will all have to contend with mental disorders, either as sufferers or in caring for the sufferers.

This can only be done through communicating, in an accessible way, the lessons that we are constantly learning through research and through any other mediums that work for different individuals – be they movies, literature, educational institutions, or in the laboratory/online. What is essential is that we avoid simply accepting the latest fad, or a story that we see promoted on social media. We must rely on good-quality research because without research it's just guesswork.

METHOD

We have chosen to do that by sharing the knowledge of the scientific experts who study mental health and those who have lived through the experience of a mental disorder. We have structured each chapter by juxtaposing the experts' views with those of our lived-experience witnesses. These have been reviewed by Professor Peter B. Jones from Cambridge University, who has added his expertise and reflections from a lifetime career progressing mental health research. This does mean that throughout the book there are some stories that relate to upsetting subjects such as loss, self-harm and suicide.

At the end of each chapter, we have extracted certain elements of the theme of the chapter that we want to spotlight. Finally, we offer some guidance as to what resources are available should you, the reader, want to access them. These are NOT recommendations because we don't know you, only you know you, but they may help.

There is no one solution for mental illness, no magic bullet. However, there can be a myriad of tiny arrows pricking society's conscience and elevating the quiet crisis to an audible one. Hopefully, this book can become one of those arrows.

1

depression

INTRODUCTION

Diagnostic manuals have documented the signs of depression for many years, but the reality of the lived experience is still far from clear. For many, depression is a grey area and, although we have some effective treatments, there is no single answer as to what makes us depressed and what can help.

More and more research is suggesting there is unlikely to be one unifying theory behind the cause of depression, and certainly no single solution. Our physical health, our genes, events in our lifetimes (and maybe even our predecessors'), our environment and society – each has a role to play in making depression a very individual experience. As a result, it rarely falls neatly into a single diagnostic category.

Depression is common and has far-reaching impacts not only for the person in question, but also for their family and the society in which they live. Two hundred and eighty million people worldwide experience depression and it is the leading cause of disability worldwide.

One of the issues when thinking about depression is that we refer to it as one condition. The diagnostic frameworks that define depression have emerged from well-informed clinical committees partitioning up the space of mental health. However, there is no guarantee that each of those categories can be mapped onto a single cause. It may be more helpful, therefore, to think of depression not as a single condition, but as a pattern of symptoms that arise for various reasons and that lead to depression via multiple paths (see the box on page 6, 'Different symptoms, same pathology?').

We are gaining new insight into how these symptoms group together and the spectrum of depression. By shedding more light on the links between our physical and mental health, traditionally considered and treated separately, research is providing us with new insight into the spectrum of depression and how the various symptoms group together. In particular, we are gaining insight into the roles played by the immune system, hormonal system and genes.

Some experts believe we may be on the cusp of a new way to conceptualise, and even treat, depression through understanding how the psychological, social and biological factors interact. This may not be a single eureka moment, but rather a series of discoveries that build an alternative picture of depression, drawing on what we know, but not being confined by it. Most likely, it will be a breakthrough that spans several generations and with it will come a change in how we view depression and, hopefully, better treatments.

Already, research has played a vital role in reducing the stigma that surrounds mental health. By improving our understanding of depression, it can help to counter our fear of what we don't know and challenge the tendency to see individuals with mental health conditions as weak because that seems the easier explanation. When depression is framed as a condition that affects both physical and mental health, it can become more tangible and not so easy to dismiss.

'People struggle to understand depression as they might do physical health problems, like cancer or diabetes . . . with depression, they tend to be less compassionate, to themselves and others.'

PROFESSOR VALERIA MONDELLI

'In psychiatry, we deal with constellations of symptoms rather than diseases, which are tethered to specific pathology. Many combinations of symptoms fulfil the criteria for depression, but it's unlikely that all of these are driven by the same risk factors or are underpinned by the same pathology.'

PROFESSOR GOLAM KHANDAKER

DIFFERENT SYMPTOMS, SAME PATHOLOGY?

Depression is defined by a list of symptoms or signs. In the ICD-10, or International Classification of Diseases, if someone has four or more of those symptoms for more than two weeks and those symptoms cause distress or impairment, then that person is considered to have depression. In italics below are the psychological and somatic symptoms listed in ICD-10. These symptoms can combine, meaning that there are 234 possible forms of the condition.

Core symptoms (at least 2)

Low mood

Fatigue

Anhedonia (lack of pleasure/enjoyment)

Other symptoms

Low self-esteem

Feelings of guilt

Recurrent thoughts of death or suicide

Decreased concentration

Psychomotor retardation (slowing down or hampering of mental or physical activity)

Psychomotor agitation (a state of restless anxiety that results in repetitive and unintentional movements)

Sleep increase

Sleep decrease

Appetite/weight increase

Appetite/weight decrease

Loss of libido

Sense of worthlessness

Diurnal variation in mood[1]

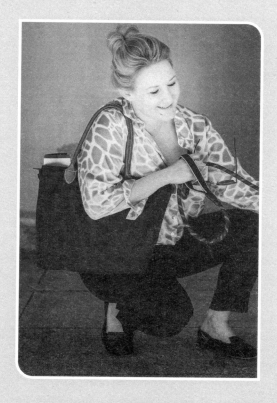

Niki Clarke founded the charity My Black Dog after years of battling clinical depression. All her volunteers have lived experiences and can provide an empathetic, non-judgemental space where everyone understands how it feels to experience mental health struggles. Its motto is 'talk to someone who gets it'.

FEELING ALONE

I have suffered with clinical depression for my whole life. A few years ago a traumatic event led to PTSD and extreme anxiety and the depression just came flooding back. I knew from previous experiences that I needed help quickly so I went to the doctor and got some medication. After that I was put on an NHS waiting list for counselling. I was on that list for three months. Compared to today, that is a relatively short time, as post-pandemic waiting lists can be anything from three months to two years. For me, the three months were hard enough. I was in a very bad place; I had night terrors, I was signed off work and I was given beta blockers for my anxiety because my heart was racing. It was a terribly dark time. I didn't want to talk to my family about it because I couldn't really bear to tell them what had happened. My sister was having a baby at the time, it was the first grandchild for my parents and everyone was so excited. I suppose I didn't want to ruin the joy of that.

I shielded a lot of things from my family and I didn't want to talk to my friends because I didn't know any friends who had depression, or so I thought at the time. I felt grotesque, a monstrous human being who didn't deserve help or happiness and I felt that if I told them what was going on, they would judge me, or leave me, so I tried to do it on my own. I really struggled.

When I was finally able to get counselling, three months later, I was in a desperate state. Counsellors are wonderful and they can save your life, so if you get a chance to talk to one, I would recommend you do, but everyone has their own experience and this was mine. During a session I said a terrible thing. I said: 'I don't want to live anymore.' The counsellor looked up at me with interest and said, 'Ah!'. She got out her pad and her pen and said: 'And how does that make you feel?'. It felt awful. I felt I was a medical subject and not a person reaching out for help. It was a clinical response to a human emotion, I felt misunderstood and deranged and, most of all, I felt terribly alone. It was a devastating time. I looked at all the qualifications on her wall and I thought: 'You are highly qualified, but you don't understand how this feels.' What would have been more healing for me at the time was to talk to someone who could honestly say: 'That is terrible, I have been through it before and it's awful. There is a way and we just have to get through it.' I just wanted to talk to someone who gets it.

TALKING TO SOMEONE WHO GETS IT

I set up My Black Dog so you can talk to someone who has been through it before and gets it. Someone who knows what medication does to your body, someone who knows how bad it is when you cannot sleep. The volunteers at My Black Dog have a lived experience and they really do understand. We are not professionals but, in a way, that makes it easier to talk. It's a softer landing. People are very good at fobbing themselves off. They say: 'I'm fine, it's not that important. I'm alright. I don't want to see a doctor.' They do that for so long and then they have a crash, and that's when they talk to a GP and get put on a waiting list. By this point, it's almost too late. Talking to someone earlier on who gets it might prevent a crash later on down the line. It's a text chat not a phone line because I think sometimes saying these things out loud is really hard, even for me. I didn't want to give someone another reason not to have a conversation that could make them feel less alone.

BACK AGAINST THE WALL: DEPRESSION, STRESS AND TRAUMA

Research has shown that stress can lead to depression, with key factors in its impact including the intensity of the stress, its duration, recurrence and the presence of support systems. For some people there can be one event that seems to trigger depression but for many there may be multiple contributing events in the past.

Stress produces a hormonal response in the brain, which influences the immune system and levels of inflammation. This response serves a useful purpose in preparing the body to face potential physical injury. However, research has shown that when we experience repeated stress it can trigger continual inflammation.

Research has shown that childhood trauma, including physical and sexual abuse, neglect, family violence, life-threatening accidents, loss of a parent, war and natural disasters, can disrupt our ability to control our immune response and lead to higher levels of inflammation in the long term. This may be part of the pathway that leads from early traumatic events to the development of depression later in life.

More specifically, if the trauma happens at a time of intense brain development, such as during adolescence, it can upset normal development and put us on a different path in terms of our mental health. Research with adolescents has shown that there are links between depression and increased inflammation, and between depression and differences in brain structure. Studies also show that these links are particularly relevant when there has been a stressful event or period during early childhood.[2]

'In modern society, the sources of stress have changed. Psychological stress from various sources alongside a sedentary lifestyle, obesity, etc., can lead to chronic low-grade activation of the immune machinery, i.e. inflammation. This can negatively affect our mental and physical health, and lead to increased risk of depression, heart disease, diabetes.'

PROFESSOR GOLAM KHANDAKER

Research suggests that trauma leaves an imprint on the immune system, even after the traumatic experience has finished. Some researchers describe a layering effect, whereby the initial trauma sets down a layer of inflammation and then each subsequent traumatic event adds more on top. Exposure to childhood trauma thereby makes you more vulnerable to the impact of future stressful events. When a second or third traumatic experience happens depression or other mental health conditions could develop.

Research on the Avon Longitudinal Study of Parents and Children (ALSPAC) database has shown that children with higher levels of inflammatory proteins at around the age of nine have a greater risk of developing depression and psychotic symptoms at the age of 18.[3] By understanding better how this happens, we might be able to prevent the development of depression at an earlier stage. For example, if someone who has been affected by a traumatic event is shown in tests to have high levels of inflammation, strategies might be put in place to reduce the likelihood that they will develop depression as they move into adulthood. This requires increased recognition of depression at an individual and social level, as well as a better understanding of what approaches are most effective at different times.

'You can't restore that time that's lost to depression. It's much better to prevent people going down that path in the first place and I think that's really where we ought to be, trying to tilt our thinking to this preventative strategy.'

PROFESSOR ED BULLMORE

HIDDEN WOUNDS

While it is generally accepted that childhood trauma is a major risk factor for mental health during later life, little is known about how that trauma translates into this risk. Some studies suggest that childhood stress can trigger an enduring inflammatory response throughout our body not unlike the response to physical injury. Inflammation is our body's natural response to infection, and is essential for survival. Externally this response is visible as swelling or redness, while internally it releases a cascade of chemicals and proteins that orchestrate a valuable response to fight infection, essential for our survival. These 'hidden internal wounds' can affect brain development, behaviour, how we respond to other stressful events, and, ultimately, our risk for developing mental health conditions.

Research has shown that such patterns in our immune system, laid down in childhood, seem to continue into adulthood. For example, research found that adolescents who are at risk of developing depression have higher levels of inflammatory proteins for six years longer than those identified as low risk.[4] This could be the biological pathway through which childhood trauma increases vulnerability to mental health conditions later in life. There may be different inflammatory proteins involved, depending on the nature of the 'hidden wounds'.[5] Detecting and healing these hidden wounds may help prevent and treat depression emerging after childhood trauma.

'It's clear from my conversations with patients that a lot of problems start at a young age so I think there is a window of opportunity at this time to prevent the development of depression. What we need now is not to focus on one risk factor, but to integrate our knowledge of different factors and merge different approaches that have previously been used independently.'

PROFESSOR VALERIA MONDELLI[6]

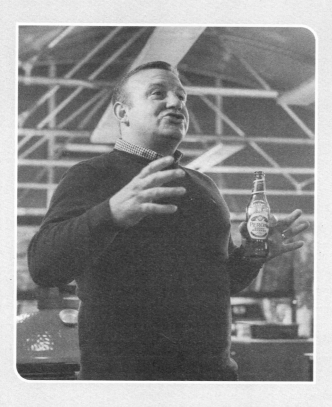

Military veteran Tommy Lowther served with the 1st Battalion Light Infantry and was a semi-professional football player before joining the Metropolitan Police. In July 2005 he was on the front line of the 7 July bombings. He is the founder and CEO of Sporting Force, an organisation that supports ex-service personnel throughout the UK.

When I joined the Army at 16 it was probably one of the proudest days in my life. From being a little boy in the playground running around with a stick, I was becoming an elite soldier and I was going to be everything I could be and more. I had quite a rough upbringing – my dad was a heroin addict who went to prison for the attempted murder of my mum – and I was always determined not to be like him. The army was my chance to be so much more. I loved it.

At 17, a boy in a man's world, I was sent to Northern Ireland in 1998 for the marching season and, as I stood there with my six-foot shield, baton and helmet, I got pulled in. We got a hiding, hit with petrol bombs and everything.

When we came back to the mainland I knew something wasn't right, but I brushed it off. I was an infantry soldier, tough and loud, and nothing was going to break me down.

After Northern Ireland, I was sent on an exercise in Gibraltar, where I was sexually assaulted. I felt so ashamed. Everything I'd had hammered into me about being the best and hardest soldier just disappeared and, over the next few months, I started fighting and drinking. When, eventually, I told my sergeant-major and operating commander they told me to keep quiet and sent me on compassionate leave. I then received a letter to say that I was out of the military, medically discharged.

That was it. My whole dream, my life since I was a boy was being taken away from me, for an act that had nothing to do with me.

LAYER UPON LAYER

I joined the London Metropolitan Police, and while on duty witnessed the aftermath of a horrific road traffic accident. We thought we were being called to a regular accident where two cars had bumped into each other but when we turned up, it was very different. A four-your-old girl died, despite my efforts to save her, and it fell to me to inform the parents. It was one of the hardest things I've ever had to do.

After the London bombings I was sick of it all, so we moved back to the north-east, where I got a new job working for a pharmaceutical company. Everything seemed to be working out. Then, one day in 2017, I was driving to work and I had this overwhelming feeling that I should drive my car off the road. I couldn't understand it. I've never given any thought to depression. I always had this Neanderthal approach – pull yourself together, square yourself up, smile in the mirror and you'll be fine. I managed to drive to work, but then just sat in the car park and cried.

Over the following months, I went from bad to worse. I started drinking, fighting, taking drugs and getting arrested. It got to the point where I didn't want to live any more. I had fallen out with my family and friends.

Eventually, I sought help through Help for Heroes and started to build myself back up and move on. I now run a military charity, helping soldiers who have been medically discharged from the military due to mental health issues.

TREATMENT: GAPS AND OPPORTUNITIES

There have been no new breakthroughs in treatments for depression for some time and the oldest antidepressant on the market is still the most effective. Until recently, large pharmaceutical companies had been withdrawing their funds from research in this field, and then the commercial focus shifted to digital therapies and apps that provide accessible support. While this has undoubtedly allowed some people to engage more deeply with their mental health, one-third of people with depression still don't respond to the pills, apps and support currently on offer.

Antidepressant medication is effective for some, but it can have side effects. In general, meanwhile, people tend to be more reluctant to take drugs for their mental health than they are for their physical health. Many feel that the act of taking a pill defines them as depressed and this can consolidate feelings of shame and stigma.

'Not having an answer to why I experience mental health issues has been endlessly frustrating, and treatments have been far from a definitive solution. Research is vital in understanding how mental health conditions begin and how they might be prevented in the future.'

GEMMA STYLES

CURRENT TREATMENTS FOR DEPRESSION

Medication: Antidepressants work by boosting the activity of particular brain chemicals, or by making their activity in the brain last longer, which can lift the mood. Brain chemicals include noradrenaline and serotonin.

Cognitive behavioural therapy: CBT is a type of talking therapy that teaches coping skills for different problems. It focuses on how thoughts, beliefs and attitudes affect feelings and actions.

Psychotherapy: A more intense talking therapy that focuses on unconscious, deep-rooted thoughts, which often stem from childhood. It aims to unpick these and sometimes challenge them.

Electroconvulsive therapy: A treatment that involves sending an electrical current through the brain under anaesthesia, causing a brief surge of electrical activity. It is only used for severe depression or depression that is not responding to treatment.

Novel treatments: Treatments in development include anti-inflammatory medication; psychedelics such as psilocybin, ketamine and MDMA; stimulation of the brain with magnetic pulses; and provision of feedback while in a scanner to activate certain areas of the brain.

A research area that is showing potential for the development of new depression treatments is the study of the relationship between physical and mental health. Some 30 per cent of all people with a long-term physical health condition also have a mental health problem,[6] most commonly depression or anxiety. However, many people with physical health problems who are living with depression would not identify as having a mental health condition. Conventionally, the psychological side of physical health has been written off as a moral failing or an inability to cope, rather than an integral part of the illness.

IDENTIFYING PHYSICAL CAUSES

The differences in how we view physical and mental health are entrenched in western society and medicine, and the tendency to view the mind and body separately. However, research and practice are now beginning to embrace the idea that our mental state does not just reflect our physical state; it is part of it and the two are intertwined.

The immune system and the inflammatory process are an example of this interrelation. Inflammation serves a valuable function, but at constant levels in the body and brain it can be harmful. Psychological stress, physical inactivity, obesity, smoking and alcohol can all increase our levels of inflammation.

Research is demonstrating the connection between inflammation and depression. For example, it has been shown that patients with inflammatory disorders are more likely to be depressed, above and beyond what might be expected as a response to their physical health problems.[7]

Large-scale studies on UK Biobank data are showing that inflammatory proteins in the blood are related more to depressive symptoms than anxiety symptoms, and more to so-called somatic, or sickness, symptoms of depression, such as fatigue, sleep problems and appetite change.[8]

Patients with more severe depression tend to have higher levels of inflammation,[9] as do those for whom current treatments don't work.[10] Studies have also indicted a causal relationship by demonstrating that when we provoke inflammation in animals[11] and healthy people[12] they develop symptoms of depression.

Research is now going one step further in showing that inflammation is not just linked to depression; for some people, it may even be a cause. Trials are currently underway to investigate whether existing medications aimed at reducing inflammation might also reduce symptoms of depression.

'The notion that inflammation has a role to play in depression has helped to reduce the stigma around the condition, because people can see there is a potential physical cause. Hopefully, people will begin to understand that there is no real difference between physical and mental health.'

Professor Valeria Mondelli

ANTI-INFLAMMATORY ANTIBIOTICS TO IMPROVE DEPRESSION

Minocycline is an antibiotic medication used to treat bacterial infections such as pneumonia. It is also used for the treatment of acne and rheumatoid arthritis because of its anti-inflammatory effects. Importantly, it acts directly on the immune cells in the brain, which are associated with more severe levels of depression.

A recent study investigated the effects of minocycline on around 40 patients who have major depressive disorder as well as higher levels of inflammation. This was the first time patients had been chosen specifically to take part in a depression trial based on their inflammation levels. The participants were split into two groups and for four weeks one group took a daily placebo (sugar pill), while the other took daily minocycline alongside their routine treatment for depression.

Before the study, researchers took a blood sample to measure the level of inflammation – C-reactive protein (CRP) levels – and conducted an assessment of their depression. They repeated these measures again after the trial had ended and they had taken their last dose of minocycline. While both groups showed significant improvement in depressive symptoms, those patients with particularly high levels of inflammation (over three times the level required to take part in the study) showed greater improvement in their depressive symptoms when taking minocycline. This was compared to both those who took the placebo and those with lower levels of inflammation who took minocycline.

The study had identified a threshold of inflammation associated with response to treatment with minocycline. This suggests that a simple blood test might be sufficient to identify those patients most likely to benefit from taking this anti-inflammatory treatment in the future.[13]

As not everyone with depression has increased inflammation, it is important to first identify those most likely to benefit from this type of treatment. Studies are currently assessing which of the existing anti-inflammatory medications might prove most effective and for whom.

Investigations are also underway to explore the development of new drugs targeted specifically at the inflammatory mechanisms involved in depression. The hope is that by understanding the role of inflammation better we will gain a deeper insight into the differences in depression at a biological level and so be able to develop more effective treatments.

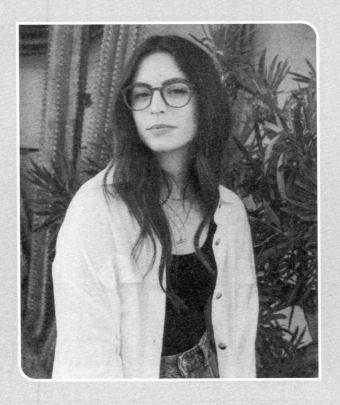

Gemma Styles is a podcaster, writer and MQ Ambassador who uses her platforms to raise awareness on a variety of global matters she is passionate about. Gemma hosts the Good Influence *podcast, discussing topics such as mental health, sustainability and feminism.*

I find it quite difficult to pinpoint the timeline of things. I don't know if depression makes timings fuzzier but for me it's hard to remember events that have a lot of emotion attached to them.

I first felt badly depressed after my first year at university. I had exams coming up and I had gone home for Christmas but I just couldn't revise. It felt like I'd dug myself into a hole – I cared but I also just didn't care. Every morning I would just wake up and cry. I didn't know how to deal with it or understand what was going on. My mum called one of my teachers from sixth form who I'd always liked and when I told her I didn't want to go back to university she said I didn't have to. It was as if I needed to have that permission.

During that time, I kept thinking how it didn't make sense for me to be this unhappy. Depression is its own beast but, for me, I was looking for a reason. So I decided that it was university that wasn't making me happy and that I would switch to do a teaching degree. And then for a while I was happy – I had great friends and I loved the city where I was studying. But I still thought I was sad for a particular reason, and by changing the circumstances it should all have been fine.

DENIAL AND GUILT

Things started to go really downhill when I found out that a member of my family was seriously ill. I still tried to explain it away to myself, that I was sad because sad things were happening. I didn't want to think it was to do with me.

When, eventually, I went to see a doctor, they suggested I be signed off from work, but I refused because I felt bad for my colleagues. I was drinking to try to distract myself and by the time I returned to the doctor's to consent to being signed off I had become suicidal. The realisation that I didn't want to be alive any more was terrifying.

FINDING HELP

I had several bad experiences trying to find help, because it either didn't work or made things worse. Luckily, I had people who cared about me and had the resources to help me see someone privately. I felt guilty about that, too, because so many people don't have access to that kind of support.

I started to take antidepressants, but while they helped with the suicidal thoughts, I never felt that I was feeling what I was supposed to be feeling. At times, I've been quite non-compliant with medication, accidentally putting myself in withdrawal a couple of times. It's not fun – emotionally or physically. But I just felt it was unfair that I had to take medication. I kept thinking why can't I cope like everyone else can and that made me quite defiant.

ACCEPTING AND MOVING ON

I think the really difficult part is after years of trying different approaches I'm still desperately wanting to find the key that fits the lock and the magic solution that will fix it. It's just really tiring. I think that is one of the best adjectives that I would use to describe depression. It's so tiring, it's so boring. It's just drudge for so long, and it just sucks so much time out of your life.

For me I think partly accepting it and letting it wash over me rather than fighting it quite so hard has helped. I think just getting through it however I can has worked for me, and getting to a point where I recognise when I need outside help.

I think when you haven't dealt with mental illness in your family it's scary and you almost don't want to talk about it because it seems as if by talking about it you make it more real, you give it more power, and actually I think the opposite is true. But it takes everyone time to deal with it, or get to grips with it and not be so scared of it any more.

But with all that being said I don't know whether people still really understand how it can affect lives. People are very aware and very accepting of mental health conditions until they become inconvenient. I think there's definitely a long way to go with practically making a difference for people who struggle with mental health.

IS DEPRESSION PART OF US OR A RESPONSE?

The experience of depression varies from one person to the next, as well as over the course of an individual's lifetime. These differences, and indeed whether we develop depression at all, are the result of multiple factors related to our psychological, social and biological systems. Despite the myriad of potential influences, there are also some commonalities that researchers can investigate in order to work out where and how we might develop and use new treatments.

In recent years, there have been huge developments in how we assess the influence of genes on our health. In particular, we are now able to analyse activity across a large number of genes together, rather looking at just one or two specific genes. This enables researchers to compare the different genetic patterns present in people with depression and those with inflammation.

Initiatives such as the UK Biobank collect genetic information and other types of data from thousands of people over time. This data allows researchers to study genetic patterns and risk factors and identify possible causes of depression, as well as relationships that might exist with other health conditions.

PHYSICAL HEALTH CONNECTIONS

The link between depression and heart disease has been established for some time, and it is thought that the relationship is two-way. At least a quarter of cardiac patients suffer from depression, while adults with depression often develop heart disease.[14]

Inflammation may be a shared mechanism and potentially provide a route in to treating both. Research is unpicking the relationship between depression and heart disease to see exactly what the two conditions share at a biological and environmental level and how they interact.

HEART DISEASE AND DEPRESSION

Research using data from the UK Biobank on over 370,000 people (15,000 of whom have depression) has indicated that there are three risk factors for cardiovascular disease that appear to play a role in the development of depression. This role appears to be causal.[15] Two of these risk factors relate to levels of proteins involved in inflammation, suggesting that inflammation and the immune response could link the two disorders. An inherent genetic risk of inflammation in people may make it more likely that they are vulnerable to developing heart disease and depression and these are then overlaid by lifestyle and societal risk factors such as such as smoking, exercise and poverty.

The research also showed that inflammation is associated with specific symptoms of depression, known as somatic or sickness symptoms. These include fatigue, sleep disturbance and weight problems. This suggests there may be a specific group of people with depression where inflammation plays a more predominant role.

Research that follows individuals from birth through to adulthood indicates that the association between risk factors for heart disease and symptoms of depression could start as early as adolescence.[16] Research shows that childhood inflammation may to some degree cause depression through its effect on risk factors for heart disease.[17]

Although the connection between heart disease and depression is becoming clearer and there is evidence that the shared mechanism is inflammation, research also tells us that the relationship is not due to shared genetics. While the genetic risk of developing heart disease does not predict development of depression, the existence of heart disease in the family does. This suggests the inflammatory connection could be due to a shared family environment rather than genes.

Large-scale studies, looking at population data from Denmark, have shown that inflammatory diseases, such as rheumatoid arthritis and irritable bowel syndrome, are more common in people with depression and in their close relatives without depression. This suggests a genetic link between inflammation, autoimmune disease and depression.[18] This is further supported by genome-wide studies which assess activity across the whole genome that have found there is considerable overlap between the genes related to depression and those related to autoimmune inflammatory disease.[19]

The connection between the immune system and depression makes intuitive sense, and it is likely there is an evolutionary rationale for why the two should be coupled. When early humans experienced what they perceived to be life-threatening events – maybe fighting another tribe or a large animal – it would have been beneficial if someone fighting infection or injury were to withdraw due to low mood or depression. This would have been an effective survival tool in terms of allowing the individual to recover, as well as not hindering the group in their fight or flight. While it's questionable how useful this connection between the immune system and depression is to us today, it's important that we understand the processes at play.

Research indicates that the twin influences of our genes and environment are not as separate as previously thought. Our genes influence our choice of environment and our environment influences our genes. We now know, for example, that the genetic risk of having a mental health condition may influence where someone chooses to live,[20] while scientists have discovered that events in our past, and even our relatives' past, can make subtle changes to the material surrounding our genes. This could influence the heritability of behaviours.

Current research is questioning the age-old distinction between nature and nurture, and providing greater insight into the assumed inevitability of the genetic machinery, especially around mental health. As well as bringing hope for potential change through support and treatment, this is also fostering greater collaboration within the mental health research community (studying both social and biological factors), which, given the multifaceted nature of depression, is essential. The more this happens, the fuller picture we can paint of the complexities of depression.

RESILIENCE AND SUPPORT

While much of current research focuses on the causes of depression, it is just as important that we investigate what prevents us from becoming depressed. In other words, alongside risk factors, we need to study protective factors.

Resilience is key to mental health. Some people appear to be more resilient to depression than others, and even those in the same family who have experienced the same life events may react very differently. Likewise, we see that some people who experience natural disasters respond far more negatively than others (see Chapter 3 on PTSD).

'So much depends on the relationship between the person struggling and the professional who's there to help. It's not like physical health, where you have X-rays and blood tests – all that person has got to go on, at least initially, is what you look like and what you're saying.'

ALASTAIR CAMPBELL

One possibility is that the layering of inflammation that results from trauma breaks down the natural resilience with which we are born. Studies looking at twins who are brought up apart, in different settings, have shown differences in the structure and connectivity of their brains. There is also evidence that environment and social factors can affect how the brain rewires itself after trauma, which may be related to resilience to mental health problems.[21]

Identifying and defining what protects us from depression is complicated, but studies that collect data from population samples over time can provide a useful insight here. As well as UK Biobank, there ae other databases, such as ALSPAC, that collect data that ranges from biological measures such as scans and blood samples to data collected from questionnaires about psychological and social factors. By comparing similar groups of people who do and do not develop depression and analysing which factors differentiate them, we can provide valuable insight into the factors influencing the trajectories that people follow.

Defining possible protective factors and how resilience to depression expresses itself genetically, biologically, mentally and socially isn't easy, but it remains an important avenue of research, and one that will require a multidisciplinary approach.

Research also has an important role to play in understanding the challenges that come with seeking and offering support. Taking that first step of letting someone know we need help can be daunting, but it is also one of the first building blocks to developing our own resilience.

MY STORY – ALASTAIR CAMPBELL

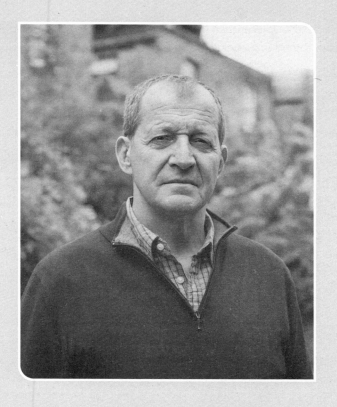

A writer, podcaster and political strategist, Alastair Campbell is best known for his role as Downing Street's director of communications for Tony Blair. Alistair was named 'Mind Champion of the Year' by the mental health charity Mind, and continues to act as an ambassador for other charities including Rethink Mental Illness.

It is a very difficult decision to seek help and, for me, it didn't work out the first few times. I knew it wouldn't as soon as I met the people trying to help me. Interestingly, though, even being able to say that it wasn't working and walking out helped me. It made me feel again.

So much depends on the relationship between the person who's struggling and the professional who's there to try to help you. It's not like physical health where you have X-rays and blood tests and other data to inform the other person. All they have to go on, at least initially, is what you look like and what you're saying.

Eventually, a close friend introduced me to someone and it just clicked straight away. We underestimate just how important that first contact is; it's very personal. Healthcare staff should feel no shame or disgrace if a patient says it isn't working.

NEAREST AND DEAREST

The support of those close to you is also vital, but it can be very difficult for them. Again, they can only go on what they see and hear. For years, my wife Fiona would ask me if I was OK and I'd say I was fine and tell her to stop nagging. She couldn't help me until I told her what was really happening. Now she can read the signs; she knows that when my voice goes very thin I'm going into a depression.

When that happens, I want to know Fiona's around, but I don't want her in my face. I want to know she's in the house and I want to know I can reach her, but I don't want her asking how I am every five minutes.

COPING MECHANISMS

The most important coping mechanism I've learnt is to tell myself I've had worse. I also have my metaphorical jam jar, where I store, mentally, all the things that are important to me – friends, food, diet, exercise, work, Burnley football club, and so on. I tick them off, one by one, throughout the day. It's not easy, because when you're depressed you shut yourself off from the world and lose interest in everything apart from yourself and your own feelings.

THE IMPORTANCE OF IDENTITY

One of the worst depressions I ever had was after I left politics, which I think was to do with circumstances, but also identity. We define ourselves so much by what we do, and when that's gone we can be left with lots of smaller identities that either don't make sense or clash with one another. I was born in Yorkshire, but feel Scottish because of my parents. I feel like a northerner, but I've lived most of life in the south. I consider myself anti-establishment, but I've been a big part of the establishment. Those conflicts of identity play into my mental health problems.

Resilience can develop as a result of how we cope with depression. The way that we manage our feelings, the support we seek and receive, and how we look after ourselves physically and mentally can all help to build up our resilience to future experiences of depression.

FUTURE DEVELOPMENTS

Large longitudinal datasets, combined with our ability to analyse large amounts of data, are unlocking the potential to be more preventative in our approach to mental health, rather than simply interventional. By following people and their experiences before the onset of depression and being more predictive, we can better understand how to prevent or minimise the impact of the condition.

GETTING SMART WITH DATA

Since the start of the pandemic, there have been huge advances in the use of technologically enabled approaches to assess and survey mental health, intervene, and prevent and deliver mental health services. The pandemic has also galvanised the scientific community, as researchers found common ground and worked together for the same cause.

As NHS and healthcare services become more digital, it becomes increasingly possible and powerful to harness insight from electronic health records. These large, detailed datasets can help us to identify the different trajectories that people follow to depression, and who might benefit most from the various treatments available.

With innovative developments in all aspects of machine learning, researchers are, for example, using natural language processing (NLP) to extract insight from text in anonymised clinical e-records. Smartphones, Fitbits and other wearable devices are being used to collect data on mood fluctuations, sleep patterns, speech variables and physical measures. This provides a much more continuous and holistic view of people's health than periodic meetings with healthcare professionals, which rely on patients' memory and diaries.

'We are used to bringing people into a research clinic once a week or once a month for follow-up. That is useful but could it be more useful to do assessments remotely in real life using wearables and smartphones. Done several times a day over a long period of time, this will provide a richer insight into fluctuations in depression.'

PROFESSOR GOLAM KHANDAKER

With the right analysis, data from wearables could provide a more in-depth understanding of depression and help us to identify particular subsets of people, such as those with fatigue or sleep problems.

PERSONALISING TREATMENTS

Research into inflammation indicates that there are subgroups of people with depression who may have different biological profiles and for whom different treatments may be more effective.

Current treatments are ineffective for 30 per cent of people with depression and research shows that it is people in this group who also have higher levels of inflammation. This opens up the prospect of identifying these people and personalising their treatment.

'There is a keen appetite for a more personalised approach to treatment because it should be cost-effective since we will only be offering treatments to patients if they are likely to really make a difference. If you stand back and look at it from a distance and think about health economics and how to manage healthcare costs more efficiently in the future, then personalised medicine has a lot going for it. The challenge is both to discover more personalised treatments and to make practical changes in healthcare systems that have evolved so far to deliver "one size fits all" treatments for symptoms of depression and other mental illnesses.'

PROFESSOR ED BULLMORE

IDENTITY AND NEURODIVERSITY

As we continue to research mental health there is growing recognition of the very individual nature of people's experience of depression. On top of the huge variation in the conditions leading up to depression is another layer of difference – our individual way of thinking and how we see the world.

Neurodiversity is a term that has arisen from the pressing need to recognise and understand autism as a difference between people in society. Many autistic people feel that you cannot separate autism from who you are, and that rather than autism being a mental health condition it is an aspect of neurodiversity. Under this approach, research aims to identify how wider society might adapt to the needs of autistic people, rather than trying to cure autism or put pressure on autistic people to change their behaviour.

Research shows that adolescence is a particularly difficult time for people with autism. A lot is expected of young people at this time and the school environment is not always designed to accommodate those with autism. Autistic people are at a higher risk of being bullied, and many don't finish school. They often find it difficult to find work following school because, like mainstream education, the world of recruitment is designed with neurotypicals in mind, and not neurodiverse people.

By attempting to better understand the lived neurodiverse experience we will be better able to inform, support, and help society become more inclusive. Having this wider perspective on how people view the world may also provide another lens through which to view mental health.

LESSENING STIGMA THROUGH UNDERSTANDING

The stigma surrounding mental health still represents a huge challenge, both for people with depression and for their families and carers. Research is deepening and broadening our understanding of the condition and of how different factors can influence an individual's experience of it. Insights into the overlap with physical health, the use of big data analytics to identify subgroups and a consideration of the diversity in the ways people think are all contributing to a better understanding of depression and the possible mechanisms behind it. This, in turn, could help us to develop more effective and tailored treatments, bringing hope to people with depression, as well as greater acceptance from wider society.

'As researchers we need to be more informed by neurodiversity, so we're actually working with autistic people to co-produce the research. By taking a more neurodiversity-informed approach to research we will achieve more insightful findings.'

DR MARK TAYLOR

AUTISM AND MENTAL HEALTH

Research funded by MQ is showing that autistic people experience more severe mental health conditions than neurotypical people. Around half of autistic people are diagnosed with a mental health condition, and they are more likely to be hospitalised for a mental health condition as young adults. This is particularly true for autistic women.

Although not yet supported by formal research, there are suggestions that mental health conditions are experienced differently by autistic people. For example, some autistic adults describe 'autistic burnout', which is intense physical, mental or emotional exhaustion, often accompanied by a loss of skills.[22] Many autistic people say it results mainly from the cumulative effect of having to navigate a world that is designed for neurotypical people.

Some of the measurements used to identify or diagnose mental health conditions may not fully recognise the experiences of autistic people, as neurodiverse people may interpret or answer the questions differently. This may lead to misunderstanding of their experience and, as a result, treatments may currently not take the needs of neurodiverse people into account. The key to changing this is more co-production of research with neurodiverse people, including the development of measures and questionnaires.

SPOTLIGHT ON GRIEF, LOSS AND TRANSITION

Transition and change bring with them some level of stress. This is a natural reaction and one that, when limited in time and intensity, can be functional. One of the most important transitions in human development is adolescence. Physically and mentally it is a time of huge change, orchestrated by our hormones and resulting, alongside the more obvious physical changes, in a rewiring of the brain.

It is also the time when many mental health conditions, including depression, first develop. Around one-fifth of teenagers struggle with depression, and having depression as a teenager increases the risk of attempting suicide 12-fold.[23]

Developing our understanding of what happens during this time and identifying the factors that can put adolescents at risk of depression is central to informing healthcare systems and building new treatments.

Enabling strategies and treatments to be put in place early in a person's life may change their trajectory in terms of mental health, preventing depression from becoming entrenched and reducing the number of years that they have to live with the condition. By shifting thinking patterns away from negative thoughts, retraining the brain and body to respond differently to events and making lifestyle changes, it may even be possible to move someone onto a different path that is not destined for depression at all.

To achieve this, we need research that not only identifies possible risk of depression, but also investigates which approaches work best for different forms of depression at different stages.

'I would never have believed that I could be happy and paralysed, especially not in the year after my accident. But with the help of my family and friends, I made it through to the other side.'

CLAIRE LOMAS

Transitions and changes aren't always predictable and, while some of us would prefer to know what was coming and plan for it, others would dislike the worry involved in knowing what lies ahead. Common to many transitions is a sense of loss. When someone's life changes, it usually means that some element of their identity or environment has faded or disappeared. Loss can encompass many different experiences, from the heartbreaking absence of a loved one during grief to the more subtle, such as when we change jobs or lose an aspect of our personality. Loss can come with gain and it can be caused by both good and bad transitions.

The way that we frame and deal with loss tends to affect if and how we experience mental health conditions such as depression and anxiety. Finding ways to say goodbye to a person, object, part of ourselves or way of life that feels meaningful and respectful can help us cope with difficult feelings.

IDEA PROJECT

The Identifying Depression Early in Adolescence (IDEA) project is a major study analysing research on depression among

10–24-year-olds. By combining data from across the globe, the project aims to identify risk factors for depression in young people – among them social and family environment, stressful experiences, brain structure, genetics and the immune system.

Based on the data already collected, the project has developed a tool that could help to screen young people for depression. The tool uses data on 11 demographic variables to assess risk, while enabling analysis of data from brain scans, genetic assessments and inflammation measures.

Already, the project is able to identify differences in how regions of adolescents' brains connect and the activity that occurs in response to threats. These differences can be linked to the risk of depression. Such findings add to our understanding of how depression starts and develops at a biological level in different people. Layering the biological onto the social and psychological knowledge may result in more children getting the help they need earlier on in their lives.

To help inform their approach, researchers are asking for feedback from young people on the tool and, in particular, how it feels to discover their level of risk of depression. Some of the most common questions asked by teenagers are, 'what happens next?' and 'what support will I get if I'm found to be at risk?' These are important questions to answer.

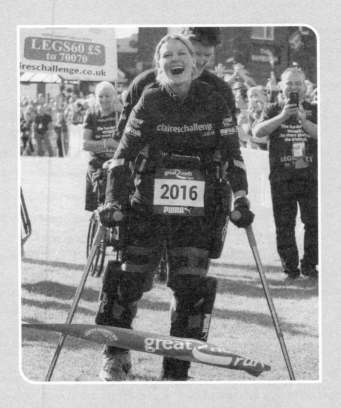

Claire Lomas MBE is a campaigner, fundraiser and former event rider. In 2012, she walked the London Marathon over 17 days in a ReWalk robotic suit, the first person ever to do so. Claire was awarded an MBE in 2017 for charitable and voluntary services to spinal injury research.

I'd ridden horses from the age of two or three, and it was my life. In 2007, I was competing at an event I had done many times before. On the cross-country course the woodland track split into two and the horse wasn't sure which way we were going. He clipped his shoulder and flung me into the tree. When I hit the ground I knew I was paralysed.

Before my accident, I never sat still for a second. I was a chiropractor, rode horses and had so many plans for life. All those goals and ambitions just came to a grinding halt. The loss of movement caused by a spinal injury is obvious – everyone can see that I can't walk and need to use a wheelchair – but they can't see all the other impacts it had on my life. Just basic tasks such as having a shower became a huge challenge for me and all my future dreams were gone.

TURNING IT AROUND

Getting through those early days was really difficult and at the time I thought that this was life from now on – the struggle of everyday stuff that I used to take for granted. Gradually, though, over time, I found there were still things I could do and the good days eventually outweighed the bad ones.

In 2012 I walked the London Marathon. I find walking in the exoskeleton incredibly tough with no movement or sensation from the chest down. It took me 17 days in this bionic suit that works by shifting my pelvis for each step. I had to concentrate all the time as I have no idea where my legs are unless I am looking down, and need to get the timing right as to when I should use my crutches to shift my weight, but the sense of achievement was fantastic.

Now, I ride motorbikes on track days, I'm planning to do a lap of the Isle of Man TT and I recently qualified as a pilot. I do lots of different things. I've organised and taken part in events for charity, raising over £850,000, and have a career as a motivational speaker – something I would have hated to do before and now love. It's totally changed my life but weirdly in a good way. I would never have said this in the first year. I would never have believed that I could be happy and paralysed. I couldn't see that was possible but with perseverance and the help of my family and friends I managed to come through the other side.

I always used to feel really guilty if I felt down, but I know now it's part of grieving and getting over the loss. The people around you are so important in this process – I had a lot of friends in my sport that were of the same mindset and they have stuck by me. It's not changed the relationship between us and it was important I remained the same person who they were friends with.

BEREAVEMENT

The loss of someone close is one of the most difficult events in life and can trigger depression,[24] anxiety[25] and other mental health conditions. Perhaps the best-known model of grief was developed by psychiatrist Elisabeth Kübler-Ross, based on her work with terminally ill patients. Kübler-Ross identified five stages of grief as being important in coping with change, loss or shock. These were laid out in the now famous Denial, Anger, Bargaining, Depression, Acceptance (DABDA) pattern.

These stages are not linear, do not necessarily happen in a set order, and not everyone experiences every one, or even any one. Since its inception in the 1960s, this model has been adjusted and applied to transitions that involve other forms of loss and change, such as injury in sportspeople.[26] Its stages are enduring in the western psyche and are often referred to in the common culture. Although there has been criticism of the model over the years, it still provides some people with a meaningful way to understand and navigate their grief.

Most people experiencing normal grief and bereavement have a period of sorrow, numbness, and often guilt and anger. For many, these feelings ease, and it can become possible to accept loss and move forward. For others, however, the feelings don't improve, and when this happens it is described as 'complicated grief', where painful emotions are long-lasting and severe.

Researchers have investigated the possible factors that could influence grief, its complexity and its relationship with mental health conditions. Several studies looking at the grief of families of cancer patients have found that females tend to show stronger grief reactions than males, and that the level of grief increases with age. People who have lost a younger family member tend to experience more intense grief.[27] Further research looking specifically at grief in those who have lost a child suggests that they experience more intense grief than other bereaved groups, including feelings of self-blame and thoughts about suicide.[28]

REPRESENTATIONS OF GRIEF

The 'Growing around Grief' model was created by a counsellor after speaking to a client about the death of her child. The woman said that, at first, grief filled every part of her life and was all-consuming. While she had thought that the grief would get smaller over time, it remained just as big, while her life grew around it. There were times when she felt the grief as intensely as when her child had first died, and others when she felt she lived her life in the space outside the grief.

The 'ball in the box' analogy of grief helps to explain how feelings of grief can change over time and continue to be triggered. In this analogy, grief is represented by a ball in a box with a pain button on one side. In the early stages, the grief ball is very big and it's impossible for it to move in the box without hitting the pain button. It hits the button over and over again, sometimes so much that it feels out of control. As time goes by, the ball gets smaller. It doesn't disappear completely and when it hits the pain

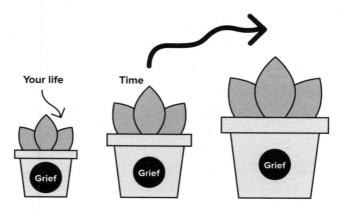

GROWING AROUND THE GRIEF MODEL

button, it's just as painful. However, it's easier to get through each day. This analogy can be helpful in allowing people to describe how they are feeling. Some days the ball is really big, endlessly hitting the button, while on others it gets smaller again.

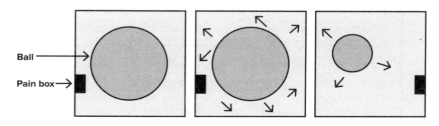

BALL IN THE BOX ANALOGY OF GRIEF

TRANSITIONING FROM SPORT

'What do you do?' – it's one of the first questions you're likely to be asked by a stranger.

There are emotional and practical challenges that people retiring from any career have to overcome. For sportspeople, however, it can be particularly challenging, as their careers tend to be all-encompassing and intimately linked with their identities. Retirement also tends to take place far earlier in their careers.

Research involving interviews with athletes has shown that the most important factors in how well they navigate this transition are the loss of identity and status they feel, and their struggle to understand their new identity outside of competitive sport. Many struggle with the lack of structure accompanying retirement, and find it hard to ask for help, because they have developed personas that don't readily show signs of weakness.

Having a dual identity while still an athlete was found to have a positive impact, as was transitioning gradually. Maintaining a link with sport in retirement was also considered to be a significant positive factor.[29]

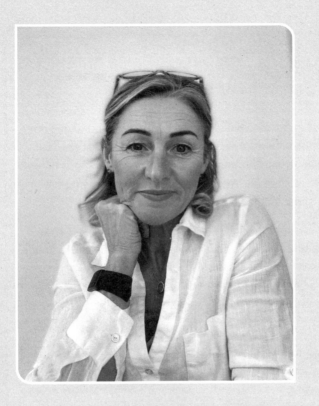

Michelle Brady was the mother of two lively daughters, Skylar and Addie, until one, Addie, tragically died of brain cancer at the age of 16. Since that moment, Michelle has been a perpetual fundraiser for the foundation she formed in memory of Addie. The foundation distributes funds to various charities researching the disease that took Addie from her. Her lived

experience provides insights and lessons into the pain endured by the type of loss no parent should have to confront.

My youngest daughter, Addie, was very sporty, but one day after a football match she came home and complained that her leg hurt. A couple of weeks later she was still complaining, so I took her to the local hospital. When they did an X-ray, they found there were some shadows on her bone.

They asked us to go for an MRI scan but, during the weeks that we were waiting for the appointment, Addie broke her leg doing a cartwheel. We were rushed to hospital for an MRI and they performed a biopsy on her leg. She was diagnosed with a bone tumour called a spindle cell sarcoma. She was nine years old at the time.

We were told that recovery was possible, but that Addie might lose her leg. They attempted an operation where the leg could be saved, removing her tibia and replacing it with a titanium bone. Several gruelling months of chemo followed, but she pulled through. Addie was no longer able to play sport, which was a big deal for her, but we directed her down another path, drama, and she thrived. The next five years were fantastic and we put it behind us, seeing it as an unfortunate blip in her life.

In 2016, Addie woke up one morning and was in a trance-like state; she couldn't communicate. She was rushed to Great Ormond Street for tests, and later diagnosed with an aggressive high-grade brain tumour, unrelated to her first cancer.

12 TO 18 MONTHS TO LIVE

It was an inoperable primary cancer and we were told she only had 12 to 18 months to live. Treatment would extend her life, but not cure her. Looking back, I think our grieving probably started the day we got the diagnosis. I went into a state of denial and wouldn't accept what I was being told. I started to contact doctors across the world, sending them Addie's scans, but everyone was of the same opinion: that we should take up the advised treatment, which was radiotherapy and chemotherapy. We did these for the entire duration and Addie was actually quite well. She would never let it get in her way. She wanted to go to school, be normal and party with her friends.

The brain tumour caused regular seizures, but she would feel it coming on and know to sit down on the floor. The last three months were very difficult. I was in hospital a lot, while my younger daughter stayed at home with her dad. I felt I needed to protect Addie as well as my other daughter, who now questions why I didn't tell her what was going on. I didn't want her to act differently around Addie; I wanted life to be as normal as possible for her.

HOPE TO HOPELESSNESS

The tumour spread to Addie's spine and she was in a lot of pain. It was brutal. My husband had almost accepted we were going to lose her, and his primary aim was to make sure she had the best time that she possibly could. I think he was many steps ahead of me; I was still clinging on to hope. I can remember feeling really hopeless towards the end.

We lost Addie on 1 February 2018. She was 16. I remember sitting with her oncology team and saying that I just didn't want to be there any more. Then a wave of guilt came over me, because I still had a husband and another daughter. For a split second, I really felt lost, like a big part of me had gone.

After the funeral, it felt like everyone didn't know how to talk to us. I must have said 'I'm fine' so many times. It was like self-preservation, as well as an effort to protect the other person from feeling awkward. We've learnt as a family over the years that we all have to respect each other's space and way of dealing with grief. We're still dealing with the loss of Addie. Even now, something as simple as seeing the empty chair at the table can suddenly trigger me. Grief is part of my life. There will always be that loss, that bit of me that's missing.

THE GUILT FACTOR

Guilt is an important aspect of grief and one that is particularly apparent in people who have lost a young family member or where somebody has died by suicide.[30] Research has shown that guilt plays a significant role in the mental health of the bereaved and is linked to depression.[31]

There is a large variation in how this guilt exhibits itself and where it stems from. A bereaved person may, for example, regret things that they did or didn't do or say before their loved one died. They may feel directly or indirectly to blame for the person's death, or guilty if they had a difficult relationship with them.

Guilt is a complex social emotion, helping us to know how to behave and develop good relationships. We gauge whether our guilt is justified by the reaction of those around us. Social isolation is known to make guilt worse, because it takes away that means of assessing our guilt.

Social distancing and isolation as a result of the Covid-19 pandemic meant social support, rituals of mourning, care for the dead and dying, and other aspects of normal grief were disrupted. This impacted how people were able to express and resolve their bereavement guilt. People were often unable to participate in activities that would normally alleviate guilt and so facilitate grieving, such as group prayer or being present at the moment of death or the funeral rites. We may well see the effects of this loss reflected in incidence of mental health conditions in the coming years.

Research continues to shine a light on some of the factors that influence grief and the many different ways in which people experience it. Grief, and how we can best support people who are grieving, is incredibly personal. There can be no assumptions about what people should experience and when they experience it.

SUBTYPES OF BEREAVEMENT-RELATED GUILT

Identifying different types of guilt may help professionals to understand an individual's experience and provide more effective support.[32]

Responsibility guilt: Feeling guilty about not being able to prevent the death or blaming oneself in some way for the death.

Hurting the deceased: Guilt about past words or actions that may have hurt the deceased.

Survivor guilt: Expressing guilt about continuing to live or enjoy one's life after someone's death.

Indebtedness guilt: Guilt about failing to reciprocate the kindness or generosity shown by the person who has died. This is common when the deceased is a parent.

Guilt feelings: Reflecting the intensity of the distressful feeling of guilt. These items include 'My heart hurts when thinking about the things I feel guilty about.'

WHERE NOW?

If you are experiencing symptoms of depression or struggling with grief or loneliness there are many ways you can access help and advice.

In the first instance, it's always a good idea to speak to your GP. The earlier you seek professional assistance the more likely it is to be effective.

Your doctor will usually ask you to monitor your symptoms for a while to help them determine the best course of action. This is called 'watchful waiting' and is usually done over a period of around four or five weeks.

They may recommend lifestyle changes such as getting more sleep, increasing exercise or diet changes. They may also recommend something called 'social prescribing', which usually involves doing an activity with other people.

In some cases, they may determine that a course of talking therapy would be suitable, such as cognitive behavioural therapy or psychotherapy. Waiting lists for these can be long, so if you are able to afford it you may want to explore options for going private.

Don't worry if you don't feel the benefit of talking therapy straight away, or if you don't feel comfortable with the first therapist you see. Finding the right therapist can take time, as everyone connects with different people in different ways.

Doctors may also prescribe antidepressant medication. It is important to note that antidepressant medication is not a 'cure' for depression, but rather a method for managing symptoms. There are different kinds of antidepressants, which work in different ways. It's important you talk to your doctor to fully understand how you should be taking your medication and for how long.

If you are not quite ready to speak to your GP and you are based in the UK, the NHS has an online self-assessment tool that you can easily use to assess your own symptoms. Just search for 'NHS depression and anxiety self-assessment quiz'.

To speak to someone today about your feelings of loneliness or grief, you can contact:

Supportline.org.uk

Support line offer emotional support by phone or email. Call them on 01708 765 200 or email them info@supportline.org.uk

SidebySide.mind.org.uk

Run by the charity Mind, Side by Side is an online community where you can connect with others who are experiencing depression.

If you are not experiencing symptoms of depression yourself, but are worried about someone who is then you can contact:

Sane.org.uk

Sane offer support for both people experiencing mental illnesses and also their carers, friends and family. You can call them every day between 4pm and 10pm on 0300 304 7000.

YoungMinds.org.uk

Young Minds offer help and advice for young people, careers and parents through their helpline and webchat. You can reach them Monday to Friday from 9.30am to 4pm on 0808 802 5544 or find out more at youngminds.org.uk/parent/parents-helpline-and-webchat.

To find out the most up to date information about MQ's research and advice into depression you can scan this QR code:

You could also take part in research. If you have not yet found an intervention for your depression symptoms that works for you, then why not volunteer for a research study? Researchers regularly trial new interventions with volunteers and your participation could help find a solution for other people living with untreatable depression. Clinical trials for new medications, new forms of talking therapies and digital interventions all require volunteers to help prove their effectiveness before they can be made publicly available or put into practice.

Find out more about volunteering for research here: participate.mqmentalhealth.org

the experts

PROFESSOR ED BULLMORE

Ed Bullmore is Professor of Psychiatry at the University of Cambridge. As a medical student his supervisor tried to dissuade him from studying psychiatry but he was determined to follow this path. An early experience in his career was diagnosing one of his first cases of depression: he was recommending new antidepressants that worked on levels of a brain chemical called serotonin and when the patient replied, 'But what do you know about **my** serotonin levels?' it brought home the uniqueness of a person's experience of depression both biologically and mentally. 'For me psychiatry offered the broadest spectrum as a practitioner. Because you have to be able to connect with people, in terms of their experience of these very complex symptoms. And there is this huge opportunity to rethink where these disorders are coming from.'

PROFESSOR GOLAM KHANDAKER

Golam Khandaker is Professor of Psychiatry at the University of Bristol. He became interested in mental health at the end of his medical training when he did a placement in psychiatry. From this introduction he felt there was much more to learn about mental health and he developed a fascination with the complex interaction between the person, brain and society. He sees the brain as the last frontier to understanding the human body. 'Functionally the heart is a pump, the kidneys are filters, but our brain is a highly complex "central processing unit" where our consciousness sits. We understand a lot about it but it's not a surprise that there is still a lot more to know.'

DR VALERIA MONDELLI

Professor Valeria Mondelli is a professor in psychoneuroimmunology at King's College London. She has always been intrigued by people's stories and human nature. As a teenager she would talk to those who seemed on the outskirts of society, even when her friends thought it was dangerous. Her interest in research was driven by the realisation that there just weren't the tools to help many patients with mental health conditions and she wanted to do something to contribute. 'Psychiatry is a very creative branch of medicine and you interact with researchers from different backgrounds because we need all these different insights to understand more about people.'

2

anxiety

INTRODUCTION

People can hide anxiety and panic for years. The type of thoughts that are so central to the conditions – 'I'm useless', 'I'm stupid', 'I'm going to mess up' – can make people reluctant to talk about how they are feeling because of a fear that this might confirm those thoughts.

It's a vicious circle and, unfortunately, by hiding thoughts in this way and failing to confront them, anxiety becomes part of our life. We become locked into patterns of thinking and behaviour that we believe help us to cope but, in reality, they only perpetuate our problems.

The anxious brain is distinctive in its biology and psychology – the areas that are active, the brain chemicals that are released, the way that potential threats are processed and the thinking patterns that develop. This does not, however, mean it can't change. Research is unpicking what makes the anxious brain so particular and how its settings might be adjusted or tuned to positive effect.

'Anxiety is like a death by a thousand paper cuts – constant small, painful wounds to your personality. In comparison, panic is violent. It's like having liquid terror injected into your veins.'

CLAIRE EASTHAM

'We have great treatments for anxiety and they are effective for about 50 per cent of people who receive them. While that might not sound great, it's actually a really good statistic. We have the foundations, now we just need to improve on them.'

PROFESSOR BRONWYN GRAHAM

'I show many of my clients neuroimaging papers that depict scans of anxious brains and what is different about them. This could be considered risky as it might be thought to indicate there is something fundamentally wrong, but I've never had that reaction. Clients always feel relief and validation that there is something they can see and it's not their fault.'

PROFESSOR BRONWYN GRAHAM

'At the heart of anxiety is self-maintenance. People with anxiety use these safety-seeking behaviours to feel OK again, but they still have anxiety. Some people are constantly just on the threshold of concern, so they never seek help and have anxiety for years without it being treated.'

PROFESSOR COLETTE HIRSCH

THE TWO FACES OF THE CONDITION

According to mental health classification, there are five types of anxiety disorder: generalised anxiety disorder, obsessive compulsive disorder (OCD), panic disorder, post-traumatic stress disorder (PTSD) and social phobia (or social anxiety disorder). Anxiety and panic are often talked about in a similar way but, while intrinsically linked, the experiences of anxiety and panic are quite different. Anxiety has a continuous presence in a person's life. It is a constant, debilitating and intrusive worry or concern, which will be about different things for different people. It can move from the background to the foreground of our focus, meaning that its impact on life waxes and wanes. When left untreated, it remains ever-present.

Integral to anxiety is repetitive negative thinking, meaning thoughts that are negative, continuous and difficult to control. These thoughts can be about the past (rumination) or the future (worry). This type of thinking is also seen in people experiencing depression, although in this case it tends to be more focused on personal inadequacies or symptoms.

In anxiety, the thoughts are centred on the individual's concern, whether that be social situations, confined spaces or speaking in front of people. Rather than being in the present, the anxious person is constantly focused on either negative events that have happened or negative events that might happen. Their attention tends to remain on what they did to create a past negative event or what could be done to prevent a future negative event.

In comparison, a panic attack is in the present. It develops suddenly, reaches its peak within minutes and involves severe physical symptoms that are difficult to ignore. These include palpitations, chest pain, sweating, trembling, smothering, stomach pains, dizziness and a fear of dying.

Individuals also feel a very intense need to escape the situation that is causing these symptoms. It's as though the physicality of panic brings those incessant negative thoughts of the past or future to a stop in order that the individual might focus on the here and now. Despite the violence and intensity of panic, some people are able to hide their attacks, so that even when they are in the grip of an attack they can seem outwardly to be in control.

'Everyone's experience of anxiety disorders is different, but they do all seem to follow a striking logic. There might be slight nuances in that one person is afraid of having a heart attack and someone else is afraid of vomiting, but the co-features of experience are the same. There is a physical symptom that makes them believe something terrible is going to happen and they then use strategies to prevent it. Because of this underlying similarity, the hope is that if we research one form of anxiety disorder then the findings will translate to others.'

DR ANDREA REINECKE

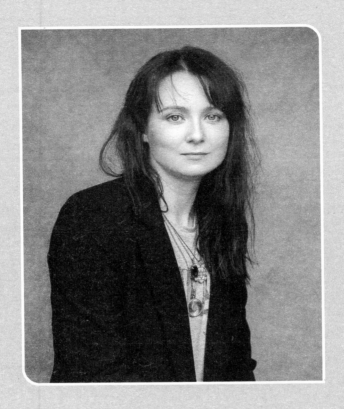

Claire Eastham is an award-winning blogger, best-selling author and a mental health campaigner. Claire's online blog We're All Mad Here *was turned into a book in 2016 and sold out in just five days. Her follow-up book* F**K I THINK I'M DYING: How I Learned to Live With Panic *was published in 2021.*

I've always known there was something off-kilter about me. At family parties, I'd hide in the wardrobe, and I hated being asked to talk about my week or do something that drew attention to myself.

At secondary school, I found the combination of hormones, new social circles and new learning styles a lot to deal with and I began blushing. Even if somebody said my name, which is still a trigger now, I would start blushing. It got so bad that I would use colour-correcting make-up to pre-empt it.

I wasn't actually diagnosed with anxiety until I was 24, when I had my first panic attack. I ran out of a meeting and down the street. I was diagnosed in under two minutes, but it was a long journey to get to that point.

BACK TO THE PRESENT

Panic often gets lumped together with anxiety, but it really is its own condition. There are many differences. Anxiety is like a death by a thousand paper cuts – constant small, painful wounds to your personality. In the case of social anxiety it's like a bully, whispering in your ear how inadequate you are. You're never completely present, because you're analysing people's faces, body language and tone of their voice, trying to work out if they think you're an idiot.

Panic, in comparison, is violent. It's like having liquid terror injected into your veins. You get this overwhelming sensation that something is very, very wrong and you have to act immediately, so you no longer care about making a fool out of yourself. You think you're going to die or go crazy. Your heart is pounding like it's trying to get out of your ribcage, you're sweating, you have blurry vision, and it feels like you're going to faint. The worst thing is you feel like you can't catch your breath.

DOWN THE RABBIT HOLE

After my first panic attack, I spent all my time trying not to have them, which is the worst thing you can do. In the end, it felt like I had to let go and fall, so that I could see what would happen. It had to be better than constantly just leaning over the edge. I found that doing so gave me back a sense of control and took away the fear. Now I knew what would happen, I'd be able to deal with it better next time.

I started to take medication and had talking therapy, but the approach that has helped me the most has been learning about my condition. I think it takes the fear out of a situation because there's nothing worse than being afraid and confused. When I first started to read about social anxiety and panic it was impenetrable and littered with medical jargon that I didn't understand. I decided to write a little book myself, so that I might understand it better – a guidebook to remember when I've had panic attacks and what happened. When you are in a state of panic you can't think about anything and this has really helped to ground me.

I still use the book to this day. I also have a noticeboard with notes to myself to remind me of what to do when I feel a certain way. That really helps me. It's almost like having my past self guiding me through.

It still baffles me that we don't give the same respect to what's going on in the brain as we do the body. For ages, I saw what was going on in my brain as a huge weakness, but now I see it as an override mechanism – it knows I'm miserable and in pain and steps in to make me listen.

EVOLUTIONARY ORIGINS

Research into anxiety disorders has examined what happens in the brain to make us anxious and has found that certain areas of the brain are especially sensitive to threat. These areas tend to be in the limbic system, sometimes known as the 'emotional brain'.

The limbic system is thought to have developed somewhere in the middle of our evolutionary journey, after the primal brain (basal ganglia), which is associated with instinct, and before the rational brain or neocortex, which deals with objective thought. Within the limbic system and in the middle of the brain are a pair of almond-sized nerve fibres called the amygdala. These are central to our emotional processing and are particularly linked to anxiety and panic.

The amygdala activates the fight-or-flight response when it senses danger, causing stress hormones to be pumped to the rest of the body, preparing it to either fight for survival or flee to safety.

In people with anxiety and panic, the amygdala signals this threat much earlier than in other people. It is as if the amygdala has a direct link to decision-making – like a hotline to a president or prime minister – and, in that moment, there is no way to override those messages. This means the threat feels very real to the person experiencing anxiety or panic and it is unhelpful to tell them that there is no need to be afraid.

FIGHT OR FLIGHT

Having a very sensitive amygdala may have proved useful in times when our predecessors experienced life-threatening situations every day. Many of the situations or objects that trigger fear in people with anxiety or panic have evolutionary relevance, such as spiders or heights. Even fear of crowded situations, open spaces or closed spaces make some sense in survival terms. While in modern times the threats related to these situations are normally very low, in the anxious brain the fight-or-flight response still kicks in. We are in a state of catch-up, where our genes have not yet adjusted to our modern lifestyle.

As with depression, research is trying to identify and understand the underlying mechanisms behind anxiety so that we might develop ways to change them. This involves looking at what is happening in the biology of the brain and in the thought processes that maintain a state of anxiety or panic. The hope is that, by understanding more about the finer detail of what goes on in the brain, we can develop targeted treatments and find ways to measure whether those treatments are working.

'To help people, we need to first understand the underlying mechanisms behind anxiety and panic, the mechanisms that foster these types of thinking or behaviours and that maintain them. There are probably multiple mechanisms happening at one time and interacting with each other. This makes research in this area complex, but vital.'

PROFESSOR COLETTE HIRSCH

THE FUNCTIONALITY OF ANXIETY

'Functional' means something quite different in an evolutionary sense than on an individual level. In terms of evolution, a mechanism works functionally if its effect or response maximises the probability of survival and reproduction of a population, when averaged across all individuals and all the environments in which they live.

The definition used in medical or psychiatric practice, meanwhile, relates to whether someone with a condition like anxiety is still living in a way that is considered functional. This definition is mainly based on the level of suffering and impact on quality of life. Even if anxiety is distressing or 'dysfunctional' for an individual, it does not necessarily mean that their behaviour is not functional in the evolutionary sense.

For many adaptations, such as the pain system, part of their design is to cause a degree of unpleasantness so that we learn which situations or activities to avoid. As such, it is possible that some anxiety responses are useful, and to be completely devoid of anxiety, worry and concern could decrease likelihood of survival.

It is thought that our disposition to anxiety is distributed along a continuum. Studies of populations or large groups suggest that the probability of long-term survival is lower in people with a very low tendency towards anxiety compared to those in the middle of the distribution.[1] In one study, the risk of death in patients with both anxiety and depression was found to be lower than for those with depression alone.[2] This suggests that clinical anxiety shares a continuum with the normal, protective anxiety response.

'It really boils down to difficulties with appropriately regulating fear. Fear itself is normal. If we didn't have fear we would not be able to survive, because we would have no system in place to tell us to avoid danger or threat. Anxiety is an example of adaptive processes gone awry, but when we treat anxiety we're not focused on causes, but what keeps it going.'

PROFESSOR BRONWYN GRAHAM

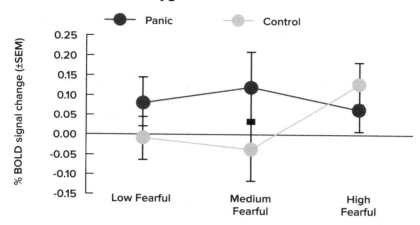

Bilateral amygdala

The differences in brain activity in amygdala between those with and without panic disorder when viewing faces with different levels of fear expressed on them

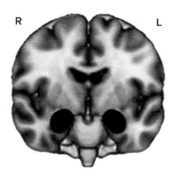

Y = -4

The areas where these regions of the amygdala are located

Symptom	Functional significance
Easily startled, very sensitive to noise	Quickly and easily responds to threat
Unable to sleep	Constant alertness
Restlessness, increased heart rate	Body is always prepared for action
Increased attention to cues that are related to threats	Notice threats sooner
Interpretation of ambiguous information as threatening	Less likelihood of missing possible threats
Dislike of ambiguity	Avoidance of situations where the level of threat is unclear

ANXIETY SYMPTOMS AND THEIR POSSIBLE EVOLUTIONARY FUNCTION

DEMYSTIFYING THE ANXIOUS BRAIN

In order to study what happens in the brains of people with anxiety or panic, researchers need to spark an emotional response and then measure it scientifically. To do this, they use images of faces displaying different emotions, usually happiness or fear. Often, these images will be shown to an individual while they are in a scanner so that patterns of brain activity can be examined.

By comparing the scans of people with and without panic or anxiety it is possible to identify differences in how their brains process emotional information. This type of research has shown that the tendency or bias among people with anxiety towards detecting threat is reflected in greater activity in the amygdala and other limbic areas.[3] This approach is also used to study the effectiveness of treatments for anxiety and panic whereby a reduction in activity in the amygdala would suggest the treatment had worked.[4]

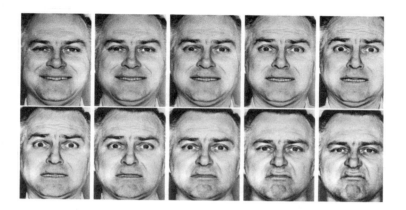

RESEARCH IMAGE SHOWING FACES IN DIFFERENT EMOTIONAL STATES

More recently, studies have looked at what happens in the brain when the emotions shown on the faces differ more subtly to try to understand in more detail the processes involved in anxiety and panic.[5] Such studies have shown that the brain activity of people with panic disorder is the same when shown a face displaying medium or low-level fear as it is for a highly fearful face. Unlike people without panic disorder, they are unable to make a distinction.

This suggests that for people with panic there is a tendency to have a fight-or-flight reaction to any situation that seems fearful at any scale. They seem to find it difficult to detect subtler changes, so it is all or nothing, fearful or not fearful.

BIOLOGICAL CONNECTIONS

Going one step further, research has examined the biological connections between the amygdala and other areas of the brain, in particular the prefrontal cortex, which is involved in decision-making and control. In people with panic disorder, the activity in these two areas of the brain seems less connected during fearful situations than in people who do not suffer from panic.

In people without anxiety, there is communication between the prefrontal cortex and the amygdala and other limbic structures, whereby the prefrontal cortex will dampen down fear responses and allow a person to engage in a situation. In people with anxiety disorders that mechanism seems to be disrupted. Importantly, it has been shown that this is not unchangeable, and treatment can restore the circuit and rewire the brain, physically and functionally.[6]

This evidence suggests that the brains of people who experience panic tend to avoid further processing of fearful faces by these so-called higher areas of decision-making. This type of snap judgement would prove useful in truly dangerous situations, where you wouldn't want to waste time evaluating what's going on. However, in cases where the presence of a threat is unclear, it may be more helpful to spend time considering your response.

Recent research involving brain scans has revealed more about the connections within the different parts of the amygdala and how these are different in people with anxiety,[7] even when they are not in the presence of a fearful situation. In the anxious brain, these connections seem to be wired differently, crossing over to opposite targets, almost like a shoe that is laced to the wrong holes. Again, the research found that the amygdala was less connected to brain areas responsible for determining the importance of stimuli, adding more scientific weight to the idea that people with anxiety cannot discern between levels of danger.

The amygdala has also been found to be more connected to a network we know to exert cognitive control over emotion, which might explain why generalised anxiety disorder is characterised by obsessive worry. People with the disorder feel overwhelmed by emotion and don't believe they can feel sad or upset without coming completely undone. In an attempt to avoid facing their unpleasant feelings, they tend to distract themselves by overthinking. This may work in the short term, but becomes problematic over time.

What isn't clear from research is whether these differences in connectivity were always present in the brain or if excessive worrying serves to shape the brain by reinforcing particular pathways. Whatever the provenance of these patterns of connectivity, their discovery may be helpful in identifying panic and assessing treatments.

WHY THE RACING HEART?

Some studies have looked also at the connections between the heart and the brain in people with anxiety. At the centre of this is the desire to unpick why those with anxiety have a perception of their physiological state, known as 'interoception', that often does not match the reality. For instance, they might feel as though their heart is racing when it is not. To study this disconnect, researchers gave people a drug called isoproterenol, which increases the heart rate (the drug is usually used to treat slow heart rate and heart block).[8]

The results showed that, even with low dosages, those with anxiety had higher heart rates and perceived their heartbeats to be more intense than those without anxiety. As well as being biologically more sensitive to a drug that stimulated an increase in heart rate, their perception of their heart rate was greater. The scans also showed lower activity in the ventromedial prefrontal cortex, the part of the brain responsible for regulating bodily functions and generating feelings of fear or safety. People with anxiety appear, therefore, to have unusual functioning of the system that regulates feelings of fear in combination with a different functioning in specific areas of the brain.

UNCERTAINTY, CONTROL AND AVOIDANCE

Thoughts that dwell on the negative and continue to cycle without resolution are familiar enemies to people with panic and anxiety. This is known as 'repetitive negative thinking'.

A common theme in these thoughts is a sense of uncertainty or ambiguity about a situation, which tends to generate in the mind a variety of negative possible outcomes – 'I'm going to die', 'I'm having a heart attack' or 'I'm going to faint'. In social anxiety, the possible interpretations may include 'I'm going to make a fool of myself' or 'I can't speak, everyone will laugh at me'.

This constant consideration of multiple potential outcomes can become so unbearable that people find it easier to end the uncertainty by making something happen, perhaps running away, calling an ambulance or refusing to leave the house. Even if the repercussions of this action are negative in themselves, it may seem better to the individual than the experience of not knowing or having to imagine a future.

Control plays a major role in anxiety and panic. People who dislike uncertainty want to be in control. This links back to the findings about the differences in connectivity in the amygdala (the emotional centre) and the prefrontal cortex (the centre for planning and problem-solving). There is something different about the mechanisms of control over thinking patterns in the anxious brain that means the prefrontal cortex cannot do its usual job of regulating emotional signals. Its activity has been blunted or subdued.

THINKING PATTERNS BEHIND ANXIETY

Research is beginning to describe some of the thinking patterns that characterise anxiety and panic as a way to understand the underlying mechanisms and, ultimately, enable treatment. It has been proposed that repetitive and negative thoughts are maintained by three interacting processes or habits:[9]

Bias. There are biases in the way that anxious people think, such as the constant interpretation of events without a clear emotional meaning as being negative. Researchers are interested in whether this is a general mechanism that applies to any ambiguous situation, or if it only applies to more specific situations that are relevant or salient to the person.

Thinking verbally. Anxious people tend to think in words and sentences rather than in images. When we think verbally it is easier to jump from one thought to another and end up in a negative place. In visual, image-led thinking, these large leaps are not so easy to make and the story has to be more continuous. Research has shown that when people who worry a lot are asked to use imagery in their thinking they are less likely to experience negative intrusive thoughts compared to those who continue to worry in their usual language-based way.[10]

Inability to direct or control attention. This has been described as a mental spotlight that is continually shining on the subject of worry or concern, so that everything else is faded out. In order to lessen feelings of anxiety and panic we need that spotlight to be able to move freely, rather than constantly shining on one place. As the verbal thinking of the anxious mind is more draining than visual thinking, it reduces further the capacity of the individual to shift the mental spotlight.

One thinking habit that explains the intolerance of uncertainty in anxiety is 'interpretation bias'. This is the tendency to draw negative conclusions from what would seem to others to be ambiguous information. This bias often focuses on what the individual is concerned about, so someone with panic disorder might interpret their physical symptoms as an impending heart attack, while someone with social anxiety might interpret a facial expression as being derisory.

This interpretation bias is associated with repetitive negative thinking, which works constantly to drive anxiety and panic. There is evidence that reducing this bias can reduce the occurrence of repetitive negative thoughts. This can be achieved by training someone with anxiety to interpret ambiguous information as benign (rather than negative) or to generate positive interpretations.[11] The process is called cognitive bias modification (CBM) and involves procedures designed to modify information processing via tasks that use basic learning principles and repeated practice to encourage a healthier thinking style.

'The way we talk about anxiety is really important in laying the foundations for treatment. I use the concept of habits with my clients because these are possible to change, which is helpful for people who often see their anxiety or panic as ingrained. I ask them to imagine they are a film director having to set up a scene to portray what is going on for them. I want them to be as specific and concrete in their thinking as possible because then I can evaluate what is going on for them.'

PROFESSOR COLETTE HIRSCH

MODIFYING INTERPRETATION BIAS AND IMAGERY

The use of cognitive bias modification (CBM) to address interpretation biases typically involves participants reading or listening to short ambiguous scenarios many times over. The ambiguity in the scenarios can be resolved by either a consistently positive interpretation or a negative one. CBM attempts to provide cues and directions to enable people to change their interpretation so that it is positive. By comparing people who have received a form of CBM with those who haven't we can better understand the role of interpretation bias in maintaining worry and anxiety.

Based on the understanding that verbal thinking in the context of worry is associated with greater attention to threat and more negative thinking, researchers have investigated whether the positive effect of CBM can be enhanced. After each scenario that they're presented with, people are asked to vividly imagine themselves experiencing positive outcomes for several seconds. Researchers have also explored whether people generating their own positive outcomes can help to improve the impact of CBM. Overall, the findings indicate that imagery and the self-generation of positive resolutions of ambiguity are effective at enhancing training effects on interpretation, rumination and states of worry.

EXAMPLE OF AMBIGUOUS SCENARIOS USED FOR CBM: THE CAR PARK

It is late at night and you are in a multistorey car park trying to find your car. You have been looking for about ten minutes and still cannot find it. You hear a noise behind you and see a shadow of something.

Participants are presented with four statements and asked to rate how similar in meaning these statements were to the original scenario on a scale from 1 (*very different in meaning*) to 4 (*very similar in meaning*). Two of the statements are related to the ambiguity in the scenario, one describing a positive interpretation and one describing a negative. The other two statements were unrelated to the ambiguity (one positive and one negative).

1. You see a security person approaching to help you. (Positive)

2. You see someone coming towards you looking threatening. (Negative)

3. You see some money on the floor and pick it up. (Positive)

4. You see that you have forgotten your ticket and will have to pay a fine. (Negative)

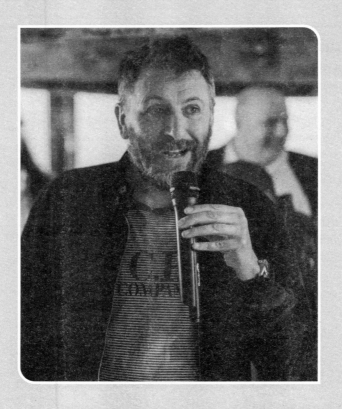

John 'Fenners' Fendley is best known as a presenter on the Sky Sports television programme Soccer AM. *As well as his love for football, having worked in football programming for nearly two decades, John is a keen 'jacket enthusiast' and is well known for the range of different coats he wears while presenting.*

I first remember experiencing anxiety after I'd finished sixth form and was working at a local shop. I had a meltdown when someone spoke to me aggressively, and I became anxious and tearful. It felt like I'd reverted to being a little boy. It was embarrassing, but I just wanted to go home. From then on, I started to have panic attacks. I cried a lot and had a breakdown of sorts. Looking back, it was probably linked to the death of my dad when I was young, although I didn't feel like I was grieving. I was due to go to Australia and probably shouldn't have gone in that state – the doctors told me not to – but I wanted to visit my sister. My flight was on New Year's Day. I cried all the way.

FALLING APART

I was in Australia for six months and I couldn't stop sobbing. My sister was brilliant. She showed me tough love and would drag me out just to keep me moving. I joined a local football team, but only lasted one game. I didn't know what was going on; it was like an out-of-body experience. My mental state was frazzled and I was crying on the pitch during the match. I came off at half-time and sat in the changing room, inconsolable. There was no embarrassment, though. I was no longer self-conscious.

Slowly, I started to feel better. I had started taking antidepressants and one day I just felt this sort of lightness, like something had lifted. I felt euphoric. I can remember vividly going swimming, being under the water and feeling that it was gone. It was a really strange feeling. A sense of optimism that I hadn't felt for some time.

ROLE OF UNCERTAINTY

The things that get me into an anxious or depressed state are the 'what if?' scenarios. I beat myself up about the way I feel, and I overthink. You wake up and that thought is there, and you can't beat it with rational thinking.

It's like having a reception area in your head. When you're feeling great and have balance in your life, the negative thoughts stay in the reception area. If you're not feeling good, though, the thoughts get in and wreak havoc, gnawing away and debilitating you. You wonder if this is how you are feeling or only think you're feeling. It becomes a constant battle between your subconscious and your conscious brain.

WHAT HELPS

I had some cognitive behavioural therapy (CBT) last year. It's good to talk to someone who has heard it all before, rather than your family, who may not understand why you are feeling the way you do. If you feel someone understands it and is not fazed by it, then it normalises it.

I am better during the summer when I can get out on my bike and keep myself busy. I struggle with seasonal changes and when it gets to November I start to worry about the winter. I do believe seasons affect mental health.

POWER OF RECOGNITION

It's important to recognise when you don't feel right, perhaps by writing things down. Get medical help and try to explore what's causing you to feel the way you do. Talk to people about your feelings, no matter how dark, because vocalising it can help it go away. Don't worry about people not understanding – if they care about you, they will. It's important also to be kind to yourself, because you can't help how you feel. I used to beat myself up, but as soon as you accept a feeling it becomes just a feeling and can go away. Being kind goes a long way.

'When you retrain the anxious brain, it's just like learning a new skill that then becomes automatic. Negative thinking habits become replaced by more positive ones. It's as though there is a T-junction or a fork in the road and, although you have always gone one way, you now see the other way. It's not a conscious dwelling at the T-junction; you don't even see the other path.'

PROFESSOR COLETTE HIRSCH

FACING THE FEAR

One reason why many people live with anxiety and panic for such a long time is that they avoid situations that make them feel anxious or develop strategies to lessen the feelings of anxiety or panic. These strategies may involve taking medication, being accompanied by a friend for moral support, or the use of alcohol or other substances to try to alter their thinking patterns. As a result, the brain learns that it is the avoidance of strategies that prevented the 'something terrible' from happening. In scientific terms, you might say that they never truly tested the hypothesis.

EXPOSURE THERAPY

Exposure therapy allows a patient to test out and disprove the hypothesis around their fears, enabling a shift in their thinking patterns. By going into a situation without any of the props and strategies, they can learn that they are not going to die or have a heart attack and the brain is then able to assess the situation differently when it next happens.

In contemporary models of exposure therapy for anxiety disorders, an essential part of treatment is inhibitory learning. This is where repeated exposure of an individual to feared situations or objects without the anticipated negative consequences enables their association between situation and threat to be broken. This leads to an overwriting of associations to threat in memory. For successful inhibitory learning to take place during exposure, it is thought that attentional and emotional processing must be focused on the threat for a prolonged period of time.

Exposure therapy requires a skilled and experienced therapist who is able to support the person safely while they push past the point where they would normally use their safety strategies. Another essential part of success is that all safety behaviours are dropped concurrently. Otherwise, an individual may well claim that there was another explanation for being OK, rather than coming to the proper conclusion that there was no real threat or danger.

'The key to successful exposure therapy is to push past that point, so that you go to the supermarket without your friend or your phone, and you show your brain that the heart attack is not actually going to happen. Otherwise, all these props and strategies will keep the anxiety disorder alive. You don't get a chance to find out that you are actually perfectly able to do this without the terrible thing you imagined happening.'

DR ANDREA REINECKE

'With these new treatment approaches, where we combine exposure therapy with a drug, the treatment effect primarily comes from the exposure component. Exposure therapy helps obtain a healthier style of thinking and information processing, and the drugs are thought to only boost this learning process. That's the nice thing about exposure therapy, it's so logically based on learning theory. It is the exposure therapy that is treating the symptoms and enabling patients to "unlearn" those associations that have been so problematic. The drugs make the brain more receptive to the exposure therapy.'

DR ANDREA REINECKE

SINGLE-SESSION CBT

Researchers investigating how CBT combined with exposure therapy affects processes in the brain have found that, in around one-third of patients, just one session was enough to change information processing.[12]

The impact of that one session was considerable; after one month the patients were experiencing a drastic decrease in their anxiety levels. While the CBT had retrained the amygdala to detect threat differently, it was only after encountering once-fearful situations without experiencing negative physical symptoms that this translated into a change in thinking and behaviour.

Further research demonstrated that this same group of patients tended to process information very thoroughly, which meant they engaged completely with exposure therapy by taking in the threats and recognising that negative consequences didn't happen.

Having identified that if the brain processes information in a certain way it is more open to exposure therapy, researchers tried to use drugs to manipulate the brain. Achieving this could potentially enable more people to benefit from one-session CBT.

The drugs in question, including antibiotics and medication to stop the heart racing, had previously been found in trials to help thinking, learning and information processing. One dose prior to CBT was found to engage the prefrontal cortex and make the amygdala less susceptible to threat, allowing exposure therapy to do its work. When this combination of drugs and CBT was given, the proportion of people who experienced a long-term reduction in anxiety after one exposure session rose to 70 per cent.[13] Brain scans back this up, showing that the brain works quite differently after the combined treatment, much more like that of someone without anxiety or panic.

Researchers are now trying to identify indicators or markers that could be used to determine for whom one-session CBT would be effective and for whom pre-medication should be used. Ideally, this would involve a brain scan, looking for patterns in activity within the amygdala and prefrontal cortex. This, however, is expensive, and not feasible for patients with agoraphobia or claustrophobia. Another possible avenue would be to find ways to identify people who would benefit form one-session CBT from how they react and learn certain information in a suite of tasks.

WHO DOES ANXIETY AFFECT?

There are some symptoms, patterns of thinking and biological mechanisms that are at the centre of many experiences of anxiety. However, every experience is individual, and research is shedding light on some important differences in how anxiety presents itself in different groups. By identifying these variations, it may be possible to tailor treatments so that they are more effective.

THE SEX DIFFERENCE

The vast majority of insight into how the brain operates to regulate anxiety comes from non-human animal studies, and over 90 per cent of it is on males. Male and female brains are, however, under the influence of different hormones. Sex hormone receptors are found throughout the brain and, contrary to their name, regulate everything that we do. This means differences in hormone levels are going to impact the brain differently. Research also indicates that, as well as differences in brain activity due to these sex hormones, the structures governing fear and anxiety may be different between the sexes

HORMONE FLUCTUATIONS, ANXIETY AND TREATMENT

Research into this area has focused on the role of the female sex hormones oestrogen and progesterone. While also present in men, these hormones fluctuate more in women over the course of the menstrual cycle and with the contraceptive pill. In animal studies, researchers have found that the ability to regulate fear fluctuates over the menstrual cycle and is best when levels of sex hormones are high. When these sex hormones are suppressed using the hormonal contraceptive pill it impairs the ability to regulate fear.[14] In males, meanwhile, researchers have shown that when an animal is prevented from synthesising oestrogen, using testosterone, its ability to regulate fear is inhibited.[15]

Researchers studying humans have found similar results; at high points of oestrogen in the menstrual cycle, or when oestrogen was administered to women, their ability to inhibit and regulate fear was greater.[16] These findings have led to clinical trials of exposure therapy for anxiety, which have shown that women with higher levels of oestrogen show better long-term response to treatment. The treatment itself is also more efficient, meaning they make faster progress and, when tested later, have fewer symptoms. The reverse was found to be true for women using hormonal contraceptives, who showed improvement, but for whom treatment was less effective.[17] In practice this insight could enable women to choose when to have treatment based on where they are in their cycle, or change contraception in order to make treatment more effective.

Most of the research that has been done on females focuses on virgin female animals or very young women in their early twenties. Many of them, therefore, have not had a long history of reproductive experience. Research studying anxiety in rats indicates that after pregnancy they regulate fear in a different way, not using the amygdala. What system they do use is not yet known but the sex hormones play a role in the regulation of fear.[18] In some ways, motherhood is a developmental phase, similar to adolescence, so it is likely there is a fundamental reorganisation of the brain towards the end of pregnancy and after the birth.

CHILDREN AND ADOLESCENTS

The system of fear and emotional regulation in children is not the same as in adults. In particular, the higher order decision-making area of the prefrontal cortex doesn't develop fully until later in life, meaning children are dependent on different regions of the brain. The amygdala is involved, but not the prefrontal cortex.

The adolescent brain, meanwhile, looks similar to that of an adult patient with anxiety disorder in terms of its connections and hypersensitive amygdala. Researchers are examining these emotions in more detail in order to predict who might go on to develop an anxiety disorder. It may be that anxiety is relatively normal in adolescence and the majority of young people with an anxiety disorder lose it as they grow older. However, in others it remains and they go on to develop safety strategies to avoid confronting their fears. Future research may be able to identify those people likely to develop an anxiety disorder early on in life and prevent it from materialising.

As the brain is in a different state of development in young people, the use of adult treatments for anxiety may not be appropriate. Techniques such as CBM will require further co-design with young people to make them more engaging and augment their clinical effects. Feedback from young people, for example, suggests that developing toolboxes of complementary techniques can be an empowering way to develop resilient thinking patterns.[19]

'Adolescence is not a quiet period. There is a lot happening in the brain, developmentally, and research shows that people exposed to social stress in adolescence or earlier in childhood can follow different paths of brain development. These may contribute to their higher risk of mental illness in later life.'

PROFESSOR ED BULLMORE

LONG-TERM PHYSICAL HEALTH CONDITIONS

Researchers are working with people with long-term health conditions to identify opportunities during the patient journey to help with anxiety and panic. This might, for example, include times when there is ambiguity or uncertainty about the patient's condition or treatment.

When researchers spoke with women who had undergone treatment for breast cancer, they found there were certain points during the day that tended to be interpreted quite differently from person to person. By focusing on these types of situations, it may be possible to train people with low resilience to interpret things in a more positive manner. Similarly, anxiety is common among people with Parkinson's disease and multiple sclerosis, where it is linked to feelings of fatigue and distress. Here, again, there may be an opportunity to tailor treatments that help people to interpret these feelings less negatively.

LIFE-CHANGING EVENTS

With transition comes uncertainty, which many people find difficult, and with that can come anxiety and stress. Change relating to identity and self-worth, in particular, can be particularly difficult, requiring a period of reorientation that can itself cause a great deal of anxiety.

As with depression, traumatic events also have an important role to play in anxiety. People who go on to develop social anxiety often faced a difficult experience when they were young. An image of that experience becomes embedded in the brain and is subsequently rolled out every time they experience something similar. Research has shown that for a child with social anxiety, an event such as being laughed at in class can be comparable in terms of vividness and trauma to the life-threatening experience of someone with PTSD.

COVID-19 PANDEMIC

The Covid-19 pandemic brought with it great deal of uncertainty, as well a genuine threat. It allowed some people with anxiety disorders to revert to their usual coping strategies, such as avoiding social situations. While this became normalised and felt safe, the fact that they weren't able to test their negative thinking and prove it wrong may have worsened the anxiety in the long run. There is concern that, as a result of the pandemic, some anxiety disorders will become longer-lasting and more difficult to treat. There is also widespread concern that young people, whose brains and bodies were still developing during the pandemic, did not have the experiences that would usually help them mature through the adolescent stage when they are more prone to anxiety, leading to higher levels as adults.

'During adolescence, the areas of the brain responsible for detecting threat are very well developed. The prefrontal areas of the brain, which help you to deal with emotional control and regulate emotion, are, however, not yet so developed. This explains why anxiety is so predominant in young people and much harder to treat because we need to take into consideration this brain imbalance.'

DR ANDREA REINECKE

'We need to think about how we can reduce the distress associated with anxiety, but also how we can bolster resilience. It's amazing that people can do so well, despite the really challenging situations they encounter, and it would be valuable to understand what creates this resilience in thinking.'

PROFESSOR COLETTE HIRSCH

FUTURE DEVELOPMENTS

A TARGETED AND BLENDED APPROACH

Although anxiety disorders have a common base of triggers, symptoms and patterns, research has shown that diverse groups experience these conditions differently. Behind these experiences are distinct biological, psychological and social mechanisms.

Women, young people, pregnant women and people with long-term health conditions are some examples of groups where researchers are identifying sufficient difference in thinking patterns to warrant a more tailored approach. That doesn't mean a completely novel treatment, but one where the materials and resources are more attuned to how these groups of people experience anxiety and panic.

There is a further need to analyse which treatments work for which groups and why, alongside an assessment of how a combination of treatments may be more effective for some. Gaining a better understanding of the patterns of cognitive processes, rather than focusing on symptoms, may enable us to deliver quicker and more positive outcomes.

There are now more remote approaches we can take and ways to deploy digital techniques to allow people to access therapy without a face-to-face meeting and to receive online support at any time of the day without an appointment. Blended approaches aim to take the best of both worlds through combining face-to-face sessions with digital sessions and support. Anxiety treatments, especially CBT, involve 'homework' or 'practice' between sessions, so as to enable continuous improvement and avoid a relapse to old habits. As such, they are particularly suited to this blended approach and researchers are assessing their impact and potential.

There is now a greater appetite for people to take their physical and mental health into their own hands, which has been enabled by a combination of greater awareness around anxiety disorders in the modern world and an increasing availability and acceptance of digital approaches. With the right resources, co-produced with people who have lived experience, people could be empowered to better understand and manage their anxiety. This should however be an optional add-on, rather than a replacement for treatment.

PREDICTIVE APPROACHES

Better understanding of the mechanisms behind anxiety disorders should enable us to identify those most at risk, enabling earlier intervention and prevention. Research is examining the possible role of neuropeptides in identifying people who may go on to develop anxiety. Neuropeptides are small proteins in the brain that are involved in determining the strength of the communication signals between brain cells. Research using saliva samples has shown that people with low levels of specific neuropeptides (such as FG2) are more likely to develop an anxiety disorder than those with high levels.[20]

One such marker in the saliva will not on its own be able to predict the risk of developing anxiety. It is, however, a start. A combination of markers, reflecting the complex mechanisms at work, will be required. To inform this, we need a more detailed understanding of how the anxious brain functions and, in particular, the mechanisms behind the relationship between amygdala activity and prefrontal activity.

Alongside the development of preventative approaches based on brain biology, there is a need for more overarching preventative strategies. Many people with anxiety speak of the importance of being aware of the condition and knowing that they are not alone in their experience. This, they say, represents a first step in being able to connect with treatment.

This awareness can be developed by a greater understanding of mental health in schools and workplaces. Perhaps the next stage is to develop preventative programmes that enable people who may be beginning to experience panic to access support. This may prevent it from becoming more serious. Research on large datasets linking data from different sources is helping to identify groups that are more vulnerable to anxiety, among other mental health conditions.[21]

WORKING ACROSS DISCIPLINES AND PROFESSIONS

As with depression, anxiety is multifaceted, with physical, mental and social aspects all requiring different areas of expertise. Multidisciplinary research is providing a valuable insight into anxiety disorders, but there is still some way to go before we can translate these findings into clinical work. There continues to be a distinction between how psychology and psychiatry treat anxiety disorders. For example, some of the drugs frequently used to treat anxiety also dampen down the patient's ability to form new memories. This could hinder a psychological approach in which the person is helped to develop new, safe memories to replace those that perpetuate their anxiety.

Biological and psychological approaches are important, and we are discovering that there is no simple causal relationship between the two but an interplay. Multidisciplinary viewpoints are needed to improve our understanding of these interactions and the various aspects involved.

Treating anxiety and panic disorders requires skill, experience and understanding. It entails challenging embedded behaviours and, where exposure therapy is used, remaining steady when someone is confronting their fears. Unsurprisingly, clinicians can be reluctant to work with exposure therapy, because at a human level and in the short term it may feel cruel or upsetting. More training would therefore be beneficial so that clinicians fully understand the potential outcomes of this treatment and the reasons behind each step taken. Alongside this an increase in clinicians researching this area would be valuable, both so they can understand the mechanisms behind the rationale of treatments and to bring their constructive insight and expertise to research.

'I think when it comes to anxiety we have such a great understanding of the biology underlying psychological treatments and the psychological changes that need to happen. It really seems like a missed opportunity to not be combining the two treatment approaches.'

PROFESSOR BRONWYN GRAHAM

SPOTLIGHT ON THE COVID-19 PANDEMIC

The pandemic has had a huge impact on the mental health of many people, whether through first-hand experience of infection, the loss of a loved one, as a result of measures put in place to control the virus or by witnessing the healthcare crisis at close quarters. According to research, one in nine people have experienced consistently bad or deteriorating mental health since the start of the pandemic.

Not all groups were affected equally by the pandemic, which shone a light on existing inequalities and vulnerabilities. Research shows that people with existing mental health disorders were more likely to die from Covid-19. Young people were also particularly affected, with 14 per cent of teenagers saying their mental health was poor due to the pandemic and 64 per cent saying they sometimes or often had no one to talk to. Referrals to Child and Adolescent Mental Health Services (CAMHS) increased 35 per cent in 2021. Black and minority ethnic groups also experienced consistently poorer mental health than people of white ethnicity over the same period. Research is needed to better understand the experiences of these groups in order to ensure the right support is put in place.

LONG COVID

There has been a growing recognition in recent years of the links between viral infections, symptoms of fatigue and difficulties in thinking. The pandemic brought this into sharp relief due to the large numbers of people suffering from long Covid.

People with long Covid experience a range of symptoms, which can vary in severity. These include extreme tiredness, shortness of breath, changes in taste and smell, chronic pain and problems with memory and concentration, referred to as 'brain fog'. Psychiatric symptoms include anxiety, depression and psychosis, where people hear or see things that aren't there.

Clinicians and scientists don't yet understand the mechanisms driving these symptoms, whether it is viral infection in the brain, inflammation or an excessive immune response attacking the brain. Without a better understanding of what underlies these symptoms, it is difficult to know how best to treat patients with long Covid.

Researchers have been following the status of people who have been hospitalised with the virus in order to improve their understanding of long Covid and spot patterns in who does and does not develop it. The ultimate aim is to find ways to prevent the development of the condition early on. The Post-hospitalisation COVID-19 study (PHOSP), for example, looked at everything from the condition's long-term effects on breathing, the heart and the kidneys to its impact on mental health and neurobiological symptoms. It found that one-quarter of patients had symptoms of depression and anxiety, 12 per cent had symptoms of PTSD and 17 per cent had cognitive impairment. Seventy-one per cent had not fully recovered from the infection.

The follow-up is comprehensive, with many participants having a full-body MRI scan alongside weekly monitoring of mental health and assessments of cognitive function. This detailed, long-term study aims to really understand the mechanisms underlying long Covid and, eventually, to pivot the study towards evaluating interventions.

COVID-CNS is another study aiming to understand the effects of the infection on the brain. A UK-wide collaboration, it draws on expertise from the fields of genetics, immunology and neuroimaging to examine clinical records, blood samples and brain scans. By looking at genetic markers, researchers are also hoping to find out why only some people develop the long-term effects of Covid on the brain and behaviour.

Since the start of the pandemic, there have been huge advances in the use of technologically enabled approaches to assess and survey mental health, and deliver mental health services. The pandemic also galvanised the scientific community, as researchers found common ground and worked together for the same cause.

WHERE NOW?

Anxiety disorders feel different for everyone; for some people it's a very physical feeling, while for other people it can be very emotional. If you are experiencing symptoms of anxiety, excessive worry, irrational phobias that are interfering with your day-to-day life, or if you are struggling with panic attacks or obsessive thoughts, there are many ways you can access help and advice.

In the first instance, it's always a good idea to speak to your GP. The earlier you seek professional assistance the more likely it is to be effective.

There are many different forms of anxiety disorder, and your doctor will need to discuss your symptoms before they can make a diagnosis and prescribe a course of action. In cases where someone is experiencing physical symptoms such as a racing heart or not being able to sleep, a GP might want to do an examination or run some tests to rule out physical causes. Your doctor may do this themselves or they might refer you to a specialist to discuss your symptoms.

Treatments vary depending on the person and the specific condition but usually involve a combination of psychological and pharmacological treatments.

For example, you might be referred to a therapist for cognitive behavioural therapy (CBT), which is a type of talking therapy. Waiting lists for talking therapy on the NHS can be long, so if you are able to afford it you may want to explore options for going private.

If you experience physical symptoms, you might be prescribed medication such as beta blockers, which can reduce rapid heartbeats and tremors, or antidepressants to help manage symptoms. If you are prescribed medication it is vital that you only take it as advised by your doctor, and you should discuss it with them to ensure you fully understand what you are taking and the reasons why.

If you are not yet ready to speak to your doctor but would like advice and support, then these organisations can help:

Anxietyuk.org.uk

Anxiety UK offer free resources on their website as well as running support groups, webinars and a helpline open Monday to Friday from 9.30am to 5.30pm. You can contact them on 03444 775 774

OCDUK.org

OCD UK offer information and advice about obsessive compulsive disorder. Their helpline is open Monday to Friday from 9am to 12pm on 01332 588 112.

Nopanic.org.uk

No Panic offer advice and support both for adults and young people 365 days a year from 10am to 10pm. Their main helpline number is 0300 772 9844 and their youth line is 0333 772 2644

To find out the most up-to-date information about MQ's research and advice into anxiety disorders you can scan this QR code:

You could also take part in research. If you are feeling anxious all of the time, or having obsessive thoughts or other symptoms, then why not volunteer for a research study? Researchers regularly trial new interventions with volunteers and your participation could help find a solution for other people living with anxiety disorders. Clinical trials for new medications, new forms of talking therapies and digital interventions all require volunteers to prove their effectiveness before they can be made publicly available or put into practice.

Find out more about volunteering for research here: participate.mqmentalhealth.org

the experts

BRONWYN GRAHAM

Bronwyn Graham is an associate professor at University of New South Wales Sydney. Her research aims to identify the neurobiological causes of anxiety disorders, which are the most common class of mental illness, affecting 11 per cent of men and almost twice as many women (18 per cent) in Australia in a given year. When studying psychology at university she became fascinated by the link between mental health and biological processes, particularly the idea that by tapping into the one it was possible to improve the other. By taking this approach, she believes, there is potential to tackle mental and physical health conditions from multiple angles, leading to better treatments and preventative measures. She believes anxiety is an area where it is possible for research to make a big difference because effective treatments already exist but they need improving. 'Anxiety is one of the most prevalent mental health conditions but also one that is most treatable,' she says. 'This means that work in this area could have a big impact in reducing the overall burden of mental illness.'

ANDREA REINECKE

Andrea Reinecke is a research psychologist at the University of Oxford and an MQ research fellow. Her research investigates the thought processes and brain mechanisms that underlie emotional disorders and their treatment. She started reading books on psychology while at school and became fascinated by the idea that your own experiences shape so much of your life. She applied to study psychology at university but at the time had no idea about the research side of the subject and assumed it would lead to a career as a therapist. She soon discovered cognitive psychology and started exploring how processes such as attention and memory differ in people who are depressed or anxious. She started a PhD on the memory and attention biases in anxiety disorders, using brain imaging to investigate how psychological treatment affects brain differences. From her work with patients she is constantly reminded about their struggle to find a treatment that works for them and the need to develop new approaches that work quickly and are accessible for a large number of people.

COLETTE HIRSCH

Colette Hirsch is a professor in cognitive clinical psychology at King's College London and is regarded internationally as an expert in emotional disorders, in particular generalised anxiety disorder and other anxiety disorders. She has been interested in being a clinical psychologist from an early age, and has had the opportunity to work as a research assistant to Professor A.T. Beck, who developed cognitive behavioural therapy, at the Center for Cognitive Therapy in Philadelphia, USA. This helped her realise the importance of clinical research, and the benefits of combining this with clinical practice. As a result she decided she wanted to become a research clinical psychologist, enabling her to have her clinical insights guide her translational research programme. Her research largely focuses on the cognitive processes that maintain anxiety, depression and distress, and how these can be treated using cognitive behavioural therapy. Colette's research has led to the development of a new web-based intervention to treat emotional disorders and distress, LENS (Learning Effective New Strategies), which is different from CBT as it uses brain training to target 'negative interpretation', a key mechanism that maintains anxiety and depression. In addition to her professorship Colette is a consultant clinical psychologist at the Centre for Anxiety Disorders and Trauma at South London and Maudsley NHS Foundation Trust.

3

PTSD

INTRODUCTION

Trauma is defined as experiencing or witnessing an event or situation that has the potential to cause harm or death. However, the way that such events are processed varies dramatically from person to person.

When a community experiences war, extreme weather, terrorism or a pandemic, or when a family suffers a bereavement, not everyone within the group will react in the same way. Some people may show signs of post-traumatic stress disorder (PTSD) immediately and deeply following such an event, while for others it can take years before the effects are noticed or acknowledged. Group dynamics and cultural norms may also influence how openly people are able to experience trauma and expectations around resilience.

A form of anxiety disorder, PTSD is a diagnosable mental health condition, described by a cluster of symptoms. As with other mental health conditions, its existence is recognised not by the presence of these symptoms alone, but by how long the person has been experiencing them and the impact they have on their life.

'Most people have heard of PTSD, but they think only soldiers experience it. Often when I see patients they are surprised by the diagnosis because they don't think it is something that all of us can get. PTSD can result from any kind of trauma and it is much more widespread than people think.'

PROFESSOR JEN WILD

'I wasn't able to sit down with my problems. I was doing anything to avoid facing reality, and when the quiet times came they were completely overwhelming. I got to the stage where I felt nothing. It was as if there was nothing inside me.'

AL HODGSON

SYMPTOMS OF PTSD

Reliving a traumatic event, often via vivid flashbacks and nightmares

Panicking when reminded of, or remembering, the trauma

Feeling 'on edge' and alert

Avoiding feelings and memories of the incident, or feeling numb

Insomnia

Concentration difficulties

Feelings of isolation, irritability and guilt

PTSD was first recognised among war veterans and known initially as 'shell shock'. While some veterans' war stories are now being heard, many accounts remain unspoken. The reasons behind this are all too familiar in the field of mental health, and relate to shame, stigma, lack of understanding and a belief that mental health problems somehow signify weakness.

In recent years, military PTSD has been given more coverage in the media and has become recognised as an important concept for society to understand. Although this is a positive shift, the focus has been primarily on the experience of soldiers, and this has led to a lack of awareness of the range of situations that can result in PTSD. These include violent attacks such as robberies and sexual assaults, car accidents, childbirth and other medical emergencies, severe neglect and abuse, and witnessing emergency situations.

A number of treatments have been developed for PTSD, which vary in their intensity, their timing and the group they are targeting. Integral to them all is memory.

THE MIND'S EYE: THE ROLE OF MEMORY

One of the central symptoms of PTSD is a reliving of the traumatic event, often through vivid and detailed flashbacks. Our brains are wired to learn from dangerous situations so that we can avoid them in the future. During a traumatic event, the brain is flooded with adrenaline, causing it to process at a very high speed in an attempt to take in all of the possible warning signs so we can learn and avoid that situation in the future. For the person experiencing the traumatic event, this can give a sense that time is slowing down.

This high-speed, intense learning produces heightened associations, whereby sensory characteristics such as colours, sounds and smells are over-encoded in the brain. This creates a strong connection between the attributes of the event and the perceived danger. During trauma, people may also encode more internal sensations, such as feeling cold, hot, dry-mouthed or sweaty, as well as emotional responses.

In people with PTSD, the association between what was felt during the event and the danger remains strong. As a result, whenever those sensations are experienced again, on their own or in combination, the individual responds as though a similar traumatic experience is occurring again. The brain kicks in automatically to flag up the warning signs, and it can be difficult to question or fight it. For someone who has survived a fire, for example, such a reaction might be triggered by the smell of smoke, while for an individual who has experienced a car crash, sudden bright lights might evoke the memory of car headlights just before the point of impact.

'I would say we have different expressions of memory and research is showing that you can erode one type of expression without affecting the other. This is both fascinating and valuable because it sheds light on basic theories of human memory and it is also important for patients as we can develop treatments that leave the underlying memories of facts untouched but remove the intrusive, uncontrollable part that is causing distress.'

PROFESSOR EMILY HOLMES

For some people, it is not direct sensations that trigger an emotional reaction, but specific words, places or even types of books or films. Some people, meanwhile, find managing their emotions especially difficult on significant dates, such as the anniversary of a traumatic experience.

INTRUSIVE MEMORIES

One hallmark symptom of PTSD is the occurrence of intrusive memories, which are involuntary mental images of the trauma that spring, unwanted, to mind. These images are usually visual, but can have other sensory and emotional elements. Researchers have yet to discover why these memories appear at some moments and not others.

Studying brain activity during a real-life trauma would be neither feasible nor ethical, but intrusive memories can be induced in experiments in order to examine them in more detail. First introduced in the 1960s and 1970s, 'trauma films' initially showed real-life violence or serious injury, but have been replaced by some researchers in the UK by public safety films. These films have been specifically designed to create long-lasting 'intrusive' memories to prevent people from activities such as drink-driving and playing near electricity pylons.

In recent research, participants watched a trauma film while in a brain scanner, and were then asked if and when during the film they experienced an intrusive memory. Researchers were thereby able to assess the brain activity during this scene and understand what was happening when the memory was being encoded and therefore what makes intrusive memories different. They could also assess brain activity when these memories were recalled during the week afterwards.[1]

The findings showed increased activation in two areas of the brain (the left inferior frontal gyrus and the middle temporal gyrus) at the time of watching intrusive scenes. Involuntary recall of intrusive memories was also characterised by activity in frontal regions, notably the left inferior frontal gyrus.

These patterns suggest that changes in brain activation at the time of experiencing trauma determine which moments will later become intrusive memories. In particular, activity in the left inferior frontal gyrus seems to be key for both the encoding and the involuntary recall of intrusive memories. Overall, this suggests that, even at the time of experiencing trauma, a 'mental scar' is being laid down in the brain and changes are occurring that could influence the future development of PTSD.

KEEPING WANTED MEMORIES

In contrast to intrusive memories, voluntary retrieval of a traumatic event involves a deliberate attempt to remember it. This is important when attempting to process what has happened, and useful when giving a statement or helping to prevent something similar happening again.

Research suggests that the occurrence of intrusive memories can be altered while leaving voluntary memory intact. A series of studies have investigated the mechanisms behind this by showing participants a trauma film, then asking them to engage in a task aimed at interfering with their intrusive memories of the film. This has been found to reduce the number of intrusive memories experienced, while having no detectable effect on their voluntary memory of the same film.

Further research into the mechanisms of this selective memory suggest that the voluntary and intrusive aspects of a trauma memory are in fact represented by separate traces within the brain. These may highlight different aspects of the event; they may, for example, be visual rather than verbal memories. This has implications for how we tackle memories in people with PTSD and, based on these findings, researchers have developed a new approach to prevent intrusive memories being laid down, without erasing or removing voluntary ones.

This approach could also be used in other areas. Intrusive imagery is increasingly being recognised as a means of helping people with conditions such as anxiety, extreme changes in mood and low threshold for pain.

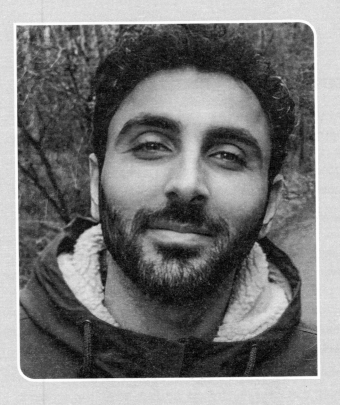

Yasar Nassif is a doctor working in the UK, devoting his life to looking after the needs of others. He originally studied medicine in Syria but following the war escaped to the UK with nothing more than a backpack. On moving to England he had to learn English and re-register as a doctor before he could practise *medicine, all while facing racism, isolation and symptoms of PTSD.*

I grew up in Syria in a nice family with two brothers. My dad owned a private hospital and the plan for me was to study medicine and become a doctor. Then the war started. We kept thinking this isn't happening, we kept saying Syria is a safe place, but the war got closer and closer.

START OF THE WAR

One day I was driving to the hospital and I passed the last military checkpoint. It was my normal route that I'd drive every day. I saw a few people standing in the street with AK47s and they started shooting at my car. I got hit by shrapnel in my left tibia but I carried on driving.

I don't remember much about the journey to the hospital but I do remember that I had a packet of Tic Tacs in the car and I ate the whole box because I didn't want to become hypoglycaemic. Even today I hate Tic Tacs – the taste of them and the sound when someone shakes the box.

When I arrived at the hospital my leg wound was cleaned, I was given antibiotics and then I was sent home. That was my last day as a doctor back home in Syria. A few months later I travelled to the UK.

GETTING TO THE UK

We were all trying to find ways to leave the country and when I got my visa I came to the UK with just a backpack. I didn't speak English and I had no money. My elder brother was also here and when I was with him on the way to the DIY shop I got hit by a car. That was my third day in the UK.

I had brain concussion, so I had to stay indoors. I was living in a tiny apartment and I remember feeling so confined. Normally I'm a social person and dislike being on my own. I still hate being in rooms like that – they make me feel claustrophobic and anxious.

When I recovered I started looking for a job. It was difficult because although I have a bachelor's degree in medicine I didn't speak the language or have the money to pass the tests to get my GMC registration. So I found a job as a security guy.

The people I worked with were racist and it made me realise that I was a refugee and many people looked down at me because of this. It was a shock and it was hard to realise that people could think and say these horrible things for no reason but because of where you have come from.

NEWS FROM HOME

Eventually I got a job helping a consultant. I enjoyed the job and it was closer to what I was qualified to do. One day I heard the news that there had been an explosion next to my house in Syria. I knew this was the route that my dad took every day to work. I tried to call him but I couldn't get through, and I couldn't reach my mum. I started panicking and I couldn't focus on work. When I tried explaining to the consultant I just started crying. I was so scared and I didn't know what to do. Everyone at work was very understanding and a few hours later my mum called to tell me my dad was OK. I felt relieved but I had still had this constant fear about what might happen next.

I have been very lucky to meet supportive people during my journey. And this has helped me to find meaning in my life again and to cope. People have helped me get my licence to practise and I have started to climb the career ladder. And although there are still challenges I feel fortunate to have been given the opportunity.

STUCK ON REPEAT

Traumatic memories tend to be triggered easily, due to the strength of the association that forms at the time of the trauma between the individual's sensations and the event. In the aftermath, the level of unwanted memories is normal, but for some people the memories continue and, when they are frequent, they can become debilitating. When this happens, people naturally try to push the painful memories away or avoid situations that might trigger them. If these situations can't be avoided, the individual may engage in safety-seeking behaviours, such as driving very slowly, or needing to be accompanied when going back to the location of the traumatic event.

Unfortunately, while avoiding triggers and submerging painful memories may feel helpful, it maintains the strong association between the details of the event and danger. The brain has a natural capacity to update the meaning or interpretation of an event, enabling us to adapt and behave appropriately in a changing environment. In the case of PTSD, however, the strength of the association is so strong that it disrupts this normal process.

To take the example of someone who is injured in a car accident: if they recover and start to drive again their memories are updated; they learn that being in a car does not need to be associated automatically with danger. If, however, the person does not get back behind the wheel after the accident, or drives very slowly, the memory remains over-encoded with the sensations experienced at the time of the accident. The strong association with danger remains and they find it difficult to update their memories; driving a car remains linked with the injury and the change to their life. The memory continues to pause at that moment and does not progress or become linked to new information or memories about driving, making it persistently upsetting.

'These memories that keep returning are not facts or figures – they don't use verbal language. They are mental images, sensory representations of the world that help the brain encapsulate what happened in that particular moment of danger. By bringing back this instant compressed picture at a time of danger the brain is trying to look after us and say, "Don't do this again, watch out." For many people these pictures slowly fade but for a substantial number of people they don't, and they find it hard to learn that they are safe again.'

PROFESSOR EMILY HOLMES

AVOIDANCE AND DISTRACTION

Within minutes of exposure to a traumatic event there is an increase in the level of endorphins in the brain. This is one of the chemicals that help us to feel happy, so it numbs the emotional and physical pain of the event. Gradually, however, the endorphin levels decrease.[2] People with PTSD may subsequently turn to alcohol[3] and other mood-enhancing drugs to increase their endorphin levels and, over time, may come to rely on drugs to relieve all of their feelings of depression, anxiety and irritability. Research has shown that out of 196 men and women who were treated as inpatients for alcohol dependence, 55 per cent had a history of childhood trauma.[4]

Some people use alcohol and drugs to avoid thinking about their trauma, and as a result it remains embedded and connected to those feelings of danger and fear. They may find it difficult to distinguish between past memories and present experiences, reacting with fear, anxiety and stress to things that remind them of past trauma.

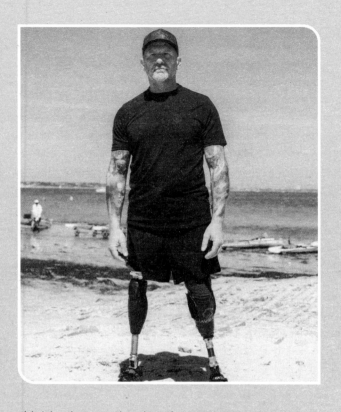

Al Hodgson is the first person ever to learn to skydive, post-injury, after becoming a double amputee. He has represented Great Britain at the World Skydiving Championships multiple times, winning three medals, in addition to six national gold medals in freestyle skydiving with his teammate and wife Pixie.

I left home at 19 to join the Parachute Regiment and my first posting was an emergency tour in Northern Ireland. Six weeks in, I stepped on an improvised explosive device placed by terrorists. I owe my life to the guys who were with me; despite the huge risk of there being a secondary device they stayed with me and kept me alive long enough for a helicopter to take me to hospital, where I was placed in a coma.

I lost both legs, had 17 fractures to the pelvis, abdominal lacerations and a broken left arm. I severed the tendons to my left hand and had a cavity inside my body from the shock of the explosion.

HEALING AND COUNSELLING

After a lot of surgery to stop internal bleeding, and considerable plastic surgery, it wasn't until the year before the pandemic that I had what I hoped was my final surgery.

Three months after the accident I did see a psychiatrist but I felt so terrible afterwards that I decided not to carry on. Looking back, I wish someone had been there with me to encourage me to stick with it. All I knew was that it made me feel bad to talk about it and I didn't want to feel bad. All I did was one session.

FINDING DISTRACTIONS

Since the incident, I've been constantly looking for ways to fill the void. I did a lot of outdoor pursuits and then discovered skydiving in March 2000 and I did most of my 8,000 jumps in the first 10 years. I started competing with my wife and we formed a freestyle skydiving team. We became British champions, winning three medals at international level. I think I was chasing that self-image of being a strong active person when in fact that wasn't me any more. For a long time, skydiving was a distraction, because I didn't want to accept the body I was in, but I wasn't taking care of myself. I was using alcohol and other recreational drugs, anything to avoid facing reality and sitting with my problems. I had a lot of fun during that period, but the quiet times were completely overwhelming.

Then I got to a stage where I felt nothing. It was weird, but I couldn't get stimulation from anything. It was as if there was nothing inside me. I didn't care about myself and my own safety. I didn't really care about anyone or anything. I was only feeling two emotions – sadness and anger – and all I was interested in was finding ways to make myself numb to them. It was a horrible place to be. Finally, I realised I needed to do something. I wasn't willing to live the rest of my life not really feeling anything.

I went and talked to my consultant at the prosthetic centre who I've known for 15 years and we've been through a lot together. He suggested I see a professional.

GETTING A DIAGNOSIS

After a psychological assessment, I was diagnosed with PTSD. I realise now that I'd had the symptoms for years but didn't recognise them. I can be staring out the window for hours and lose connection with my senses, time and who I am, something called 'dissociation'. I also have hyperarousal, common in PTSD, where I am constantly irritable, angry and startled by certain things. I always thought that I had a short fuse, but when I think back to those times when I have gone from 0 to 10 with anger, it's not normal or acceptable.

ACCEPTANCE AND SUPPORT

When I thought of PTSD I imagined somebody cowering in the corner when they heard a loud bang or being anxious about everything. Maybe they are symptoms for some people, but for me there's guilt involved and I often wish I had never woken up.

It's a real palpable fear that I don't know how I will get through the day and that something terrible could happen at any given moment.

It's only now I can understand why some people can't get out of bed in the morning. In the past I might have thought, 'What do you mean? Just get out of bed!' But now I can see that's the only place where they're going to feel safe.

I think if it wasn't for my wife I would still be taking drugs and drinking a lot. She confronted me with the person I'd become and, as a result, a new emotion was born: embarrassment. Although that wasn't comfortable, it told me that I do care about other people.

OTHER MEMORY PROBLEMS

As well as causing recurring memories of the trauma itself, PTSD can impact on the mind's ability to store, recall and synthesise memories of events thereafter. This makes sense: when your brain is full of highly encoded trauma memories there simply isn't the same capacity for concentration or short-term memory.

Given that PTSD can also impact negatively on sleep (due again to recurrent memories), this can further reduce the individual's ability to remember. Research has demonstrated that people with PTSD who perform worse on memory tasks also find therapy less effective. It seems they can't update those memories that are so heavily imprinted with emotion, and this impacts more generally on their memory skills.

Research has also shown that people with PTSD are more likely to develop Alzheimer's disease in later life. The exact reasons for this are unknown, and it is not clear whether a predisposition to PTSD is also a predisposition to Alzheimer's, or if PTSD functions as a risk factor. In some populations, the risk of Alzheimer's is twice as high among people with a PTSD diagnosis.[5] This suggests that the mental processes involved in PTSD may also be involved in dementia, and the loss of memory in both may be linked.

At times, PTSD can create symptoms similar to those of ADHD, which can compound memory problems further and make it more difficult to learn or take in new information. This process is thought to originate from the same brain mechanisms that regulate mood and synthesise information, which may be why mood, cognition and memory are all impaired by post-traumatic stress. Researchers are investigating the overlap between ADHD and PTSD to try to identify possible shared mechanisms that could help in treatment.[6]

Crucial to treatment is helping people to update the meaning of their memories and break the links between past trauma and present experience. However, due to the general memory problems and avoidance behaviour that result from PTSD, there are a number of barriers to this process.

One approach is to teach people that the memories they have aren't dangerous, and therefore don't need to be pushed away or dwelled upon. As well as helping people to tolerate their memories, this enables them to engage more fully in their lives without avoiding situations that they believe will cause anxiety.

PREDICTING VULNERABILITY TO PTSD

Everyone's experience of PTSD is different and some people are more likely to develop the condition than others. Poor sleep, memory suppression, negative thinking and alcohol use all increase the likelihood that someone will develop PTSD.

Dwelling on, or overthinking, past events is also a key factor. In many ways dwelling is a form of avoidance, as it doesn't allow the individual to update their memories and move on.

A tendency to think visually has also been proposed as contributing to the development of PTSD. Those with strong visualisation skills are likely to have memories that are more detailed, more intense and potentially more difficult to reframe. These are often found in people with mental health conditions such as bipolar disorder and autism spectrum disorder, and these groups have been found to be more at risk of PTSD.

'I want people to recognise how harmful "dwelling" is as a thinking style because it's not actually helping us to solve problems or think more clearly or find a solution. It keeps us in our head and prevents processing, so it's important that we disengage with it as quickly as possible.'

PROFESSOR JENNIFER WILD

'We know that emergency workers will be exposed to horrible stuff in their occupational lives, but also in their personal lives they have a high rate of trauma. We know that this predicts PTSD, so we can develop a preventative intervention. We've been able to reduce episodes of PTSD and depression in student paramedics, who we've trained to disengage from dwelling in their thinking.'

PROFESSOR JENNIFER WILD

RISK FACTORS FOR PTSD IN PARAMEDICS

In one study, psychological and personality assessments were made of around 400 paramedics to gain a detailed picture on how they think and behave. Researchers then assessed them for exposure to trauma and PTSD symptoms every four months for two years.[7] It was found that only one factor, dwelling, predicted PTSD, while having a negative view of their own resilience was also more common in those who developed PTSD. This relationship was found even when controlling for severity of the trauma and past psychological problems. This insight is potentially useful in the development of more targeted and pre-emptive support, particularly for people who are likely to experience trauma often, for example those in occupations such as paramedic, who experience many distressing events in their work.

Researchers, for example, have developed internet-based support that combines existing therapies for PTSD with new approaches aimed at helping people to stop dwelling on negative thoughts. As part of this, individuals are provided with reminders of what they have learnt to reinforce the impact of the therapy. Researchers are evaluating the approach using student paramedics, some of whom will follow the new support programme, while others will use existing online support. Others will receive no special support at all. The results should indicate whether upfront training can prevent depression and PTSD from becoming serious problems.[8]

It has been proposed that there are three possible outcomes after trauma: the individual either carries on as usual, goes on to thrive, or develops PTSD. Typically, researchers haven't studied those people who go on to thrive or carry on with their lives post-trauma, but it is an emerging field.

There may be ways of thinking and behaviours that make us more resilient to trauma. Some research suggests that the experience of trauma may switch on a resilient gene or group of genes, which means we're better able to cope with trauma in the future. A review of research in this area identified six genes associated with psychological resilience.[9] Evidence also indicates, however, that whether this genetic resilience prevents trauma translating into PTSD is strongly influenced by factors such as sex, ethnic background and socioeconomic status, as well as modifiable predictors such as dwelling as a thinking style, rumination and a neurotic personality.

CUMULATIVE TRAUMA

Around one-third of people who experience something traumatic will develop PTSD, sometimes months or years after the incident. The timing and context of the event is integral to if and when symptoms develop. There is evidence that for some people trauma is cumulative and it may not be the first or the second experience that triggers PTSD. It might not even be the event that seems the most traumatic, but one that appears minor in comparison. This tallies with the idea that the impact of trauma layers itself up within in an individual (see Chapter 1 on childhood trauma and inflammation) and this can influence our mental and physical health.

Researchers are investigating whether the level of arousal at the time of an event plays a role in mediating whether PTSD develops. For example, if you have an argument at work shortly before witnessing a traumatic event, you may be hypersensitive, causing the reactions of over-encoding and sensory stimulation to be more pronounced. This would suggest there is almost a base layer of vigilance caused by the arousal, so when the trauma occurs PTSD symptoms are more easily triggered.

'In some cases, the event can seem minor in the grand scheme of things and yet this is the one after which people develop PTSD. What's important is the meaning we attribute to these events, how we interpret them and the strategies we engage in that maintain the distress.'

PROFESSOR JENNIFER WILD

COMPLEX PTSD

Complex PTSD may be diagnosed in people who have experienced repeated traumatic events, such as violence, torture, neglect or abuse, usually involving one other person or more. The resulting PTSD may be more severe if the traumatic events happened early in life, if they were caused by a parent or carer, if there is still contact with the person responsible, or if escape or rescue was unlikely.

The term 'complex PTSD' is fairly new. Although there is recognition that some types of trauma can have more severe effects, not everyone is in agreement as to whether this is still a form of PTSD or an entirely separate condition.

People with complex PTSD are likely to experience 'emotional flashbacks', in which they relive the intense feelings that they had during the trauma, such as fear, shame, sadness or despair. They may react to events in the present as though they are responsible for these feelings, without realising the real cause. As it can take years for the symptoms of complex PTSD to be recognised, a child's development may be affected, while adults with complex PTSD may lose their trust in people and feel separated from others.

SYMPTOMS OF COMPLEX PTSD

Feelings of shame or guilt

Difficulty controlling emotions

Periods of losing attention and concentration (dissociation)

Physical symptoms, such as headaches, dizziness, chest pains and stomach aches

Feeling very angry or distrustful towards the world

Constant feelings of emptiness or hopelessness

Feeling permanently damaged or worthless

Feeling completely different from other people

Cutting yourself off from friends and family

Relationship difficulties

Destructive or risky behaviour, such as self-harm, alcohol misuse or drug abuse

Suicidal thoughts

MY STORY – REBECCA WOOLDRIDGE

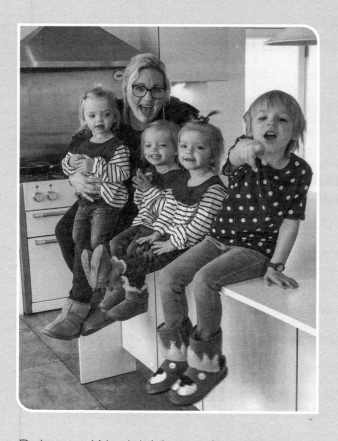

Rebecca Wooldridge writes about her experiences via her blog at mummytotripletsandbro.com and shares her daily tales of parenting, including the fun, the wins and even the fails, on Instagram.

It had been a difficult journey to become pregnant and when we found out it was triplets we knew it would be risky. It was scary all the way through, and I didn't enjoy it as much as I had done my previous pregnancy. The girls arrived at 29 weeks, when I was already under observation in the hospital. I had haemorrhaged and an early C-section was necessary for all of us to survive.

RECOGNISING PTSD

Afterwards, I felt like a very different person. My body was recovering and responding to this near-death experience, but I knew I had changed. I had three very poorly babies in intensive care. My life became about being in the hospital and being completely dependent on others.

I was aware of how different I felt, but I didn't understand it and that made me frightened. My babies were in intensive care and there were so many emotions. When I realised that I was scared to be by myself and it felt like the walls were closing in, I knew something was wrong. I didn't understand that the feelings were part of PTSD. I guess because I associated it with being a soldier and the trauma of war and didn't think it was something I would experience.

I started to have these physical reactions – I couldn't close my eyes, not even to wash my face, because every time I closed my eyes I'd get flashbacks of the trauma. I needed to recover physically, I needed to get my strength back but I was frightened of going to sleep. Looking back, I think it was related to when I was anaesthetised for the emergency C-section: in that moment, I was so scared of dying. Everything was happening so quickly and I could feel the extreme blood loss. I knew I was in trouble and I could hear the panicked voices of the staff all around me. As I closed my eyes I didn't know if I'd wake up again. After that, every time I closed my eyes, I was reminded of the fear of not opening them again.

I was diagnosed with PTSD while still in hospital, and it was helpful to have the diagnosis. It made me feel human to have this condition that was understood and logical and not just something wrong with me. But there was still so much happening with the girls' health. After 11 weeks in hospital all of them came home. Amelie was the last, and within days she got very poorly. Terrifyingly, and after just nine days at home, she was in my arms when she stopped breathing. I felt it happen, and if I hadn't been holding her at the time it would been a very different outcome. She went back in intensive care and was put into a coma because she couldn't breathe for herself and then as she came out of her coma, her sister Bertie was taken in. She was blue-lighted to high-dependency and weeks later she had to have emergency heart surgery. Then when she came home, they all got really bad chicken pox, which felt manageable comparatively, but as we were nursing them we found a lump in Amelie's neck – it became life-threatening as it was growing on her airway, so we lived in fear that her breathing would be affected again. She needed emergency biopsy surgery to have the lump removed; it was found to be benign.

So it was just one frightening event after the other. I was a nervous wreck. I think when you've been exposed to prolonged trauma and extreme fear, your brain can feel predisposed to bad things happening because they already did, and you just feel at any moment something terrible will happen again.

THERAPY AND SUPPORT

It's hard when you're in the moment of the trauma happening, it's awful. You're running on adrenaline so your body is somehow helping you cope, but after the event/s when you've got time to think about what has happened, it's just too painful to think about. Your brain doesn't want to process the memories and shuts them down unprocessed, and that's when it becomes a massive issue for your mental health.

I managed to get referred to have EMDR [eye movement desensitisation and reprocessing] through a birth trauma charity and that helped me get to a place where I could manage my PTSD symptoms. I was able to work through the previously unprocessed memories that had been stuck in a really unhelpful loop in my head, causing me to feel constantly anxious. I was able to process them like I would any other memory, and put them away safely. It didn't make the memories pleasant, but it made them manageable so they weren't too painful to think about any more.

One of the things I've learnt through this journey is to reframe things that happened. I had a lot of 'what ifs' and things I wished had happened differently, but if I look at them in a different way I can sometimes see the positive, or learn to accept the negative. For example, I had to have an emergency C-section under anaesthesia, so I wasn't awake when the girls were born to hear their first cry. But I have come to understand that if I had been awake it would have been terrifying, because two of my daughters were born not breathing. So I've learnt to reframe this event to think perhaps it was better that I wasn't awake, because I'm not sure I could have coped with that fear.

For cases like mine I think the link between being in hospital for emergency situations and having quick access to mental health support needs to be stronger, and we also need to consider the wider family. Our experience has had a huge impact on my husband as well. For him the trauma with the children and their health was just as constant and terrifying.

BUILDING A COMMUNITY

I find writing my own blogs and posts has been really cathartic. But more than anything I love it when I hear that someone has been helped by what I've written, because that's why I started it and that's what helped me – reading survival stories. It can be a really useful route to find your tribe and hear from like-minded people who get it.

I think that this kind of trauma does change you but, on the flip side, this can be in a good way. It's very empowering to accept where I am today and say that a part of me was broken by the trauma but I've put the pieces back together

The new version is a better version of me. I can't change what happened. It will always feel painful to remember, and I haven't recovered from my sadness at my babies being born too soon, but I've managed to reframe a lot of what happened. The lessons I've learnt are a gift. I am hugely grateful and appreciative of all that I have because I am very lucky to be here with my children. It was nearly very different. I don't sweat the small stuff any more. Life is too precious.

For those with similar experiences to mine, I would just say be kind to yourself. Feeling emotional about an emotional event doesn't mean there is anything wrong with you. PTSD can feel scary and isolating. I remember feeling I was failing because my mental health was impacted. I don't think that now. On the contrary, I think responding to trauma is a logical response to what has happened. We're not robots. We should allow ourselves to feel, because suppressing the feelings is unhelpful to our mental health in the long term. Finding a group of people to share your experience in a safe space can really help. That may be in person or online.

PTSD TREATMENTS

There is a range of evidence-based treatments available for PTSD, some focusing on changing thoughts and behaviour, others attempting to desensitise or make the event and memories less frightening. This works in a similar way to exposure therapy, as seen in Chapter 2.

TRAUMA-FOCUSED COGNITIVE BEHAVIOURAL THERAPY (CBT)

This approach harnesses a range of psychological techniques to help the individual come to terms with a traumatic event. The therapist helps them to gain control of their fear and distress by discussing the conclusions they have drawn about their experience. They may, for example, feel to blame for what happened or fear that it will happen again. The therapist may encourage them to restart, gradually, those activities that they have avoided since the trauma.

EYE MOVEMENT DESENSITISATION AND REPROCESSING (EMDR)

This psychological treatment involves the patient recalling the details of their traumatic incident while making eye movements, usually by following the movement of the therapist's finger. While they are thinking or talking about their memories, they are asked to focus on their eye movements or sometimes other stimuli such as hand taps, as well as sounds. It's not clear exactly how EMDR works, but it may interfere with memory recall so that the memory/emotion links are not so strong.

COGNITIVE PROCESSING THERAPY (CPT)

This is a specific type of CBT that involves trying to change thinking patterns. People undergoing CPT are helped to understand and change how they think about their trauma and its aftermath. The goal is to understand how certain thoughts about the trauma cause stress and make symptoms worse, which then enables change.

PROLONGED EXPOSURE THERAPY

The goal of this therapy is to make the memories of a traumatic event less fearful. The patient talks about their trauma with a therapist in a safe, gradual way, and listens to recordings of these conversations between sessions to gain control of their thoughts and feelings.

RESHAPING MEMORIES

Researchers are conducting a trial of a new combination of therapies designed for emergency responders, called the SHAPE recovery approach. Originally focused on paramedics, this study was expanded as a result of the pandemic to look at all frontline healthcare workers in hospitals. Exposure to trauma is common among healthcare workers, but during the Covid-19 pandemic it was a particular problem. Research shows that 44 per cent of healthcare workers on the front line during the pandemic met the criteria for PTSD and 39 per cent met criteria for major depressive disorder.[10]

The sights and sounds of the healthcare environment, such as the beeps of monitors, can become linked to suffering and death for frontline workers. The SHAPE approach seeks to break these negative associations, as these are sounds and sights they will continue to face in their everyday work. Individuals aren't required to change the facts of the traumatic event they've experienced, but rather to retell the story in a way that breaks negative links and assigns new meanings to memories. For example, rather than recalling a story of suffering, they might focus on how courageously they and their colleagues coped, and the people they managed to help. This approach has achieved a recovery rate of 90 per cent in emergency workers and, by giving them the tools they need, has helped to prevent others from developing post-traumatic stress and depression.[11]

INTERFERING WITH RECONSOLIDATION OF MEMORIES

Treatments such as CBT and exposure therapy work by changing beliefs, fears and, subsequently, behaviour around trauma. However, some approaches aim to target patients' thought processes as soon as possible after the event in order to interfere with the storing of trauma memories while they're still liable to change. Different, more positive, versions of the memory can then be consolidated.

In this treatment, trauma memory 'hotspots' are activated briefly using reminders, then the patient is asked to perform a visuospatial task designed to interfere with memory recall, such as playing Tetris. The idea is that this very visually demanding task will interfere with the consolidation or reconsolidation of the visual components of the trauma memory, targeted at those memory segments that are particularly intrusive. Using this induced trauma imagery, the treatment has been shown to be successful in reducing the number of intrusive memories and images by about half.

INTRUSIVE MEMORIES IN DIFFERENT SETTINGS

Over the years, the approach of interfering with the laying down of intrusive memories has been tested on different groups and in various settings. Women have been given the therapy six hours after traumatic childbirth by C-section,[12] as have survivors of vehicle accidents, again six hours after their crashes have taken place.[13] For patients with complex PTSD, meanwhile, researchers have used a version adapted for older memories.[14] In these cases, the approach has so far only been evaluated in the short term. It now needs assessment over a longer time period and on a greater diversity of trauma experiences.

A more recent study has investigated the effects of task intervention on intrusive memories on people who presented at emergency departments having experienced a range of traumas. Intrusive memories were assessed using a memory diary, then follow-up assessments were conducted at weekly and monthly intervals. Levels of distress and anxiety were also measured.

Participants carried out the visuospatial task on their smartphones, rather than using a game console as in previous studies, while the control group listened instead to a podcast and received no therapy. Those who received the therapy reported fewer intrusive memories of trauma at weeks one and five. The findings will inform future trials on the use of cognitive task intervention to reduce the occurrence of intrusive memories after traumatic events.

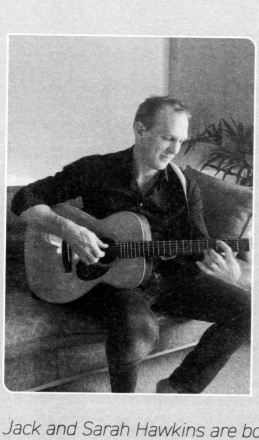

Jack and Sarah Hawkins are both medical professionals, and until 2016 both worked at the same hospital trust, Sarah as a physiotherapist and Jack as a consultant. They won what is thought to be the largest settlement in UK legal history for a stillbirth criminal negligence claim, following a five-year fight for justice for their daughter Harriet.

When Sarah handed me the pregnancy test, wrapped up in a box, I couldn't believe it. I had a job that I enjoyed, working with medical teams all over the country, and we were about to start a family. Life was great.

COPING AND FIGHTING

We both worked at the hospital where we were due to have Harriet, but we insisted we didn't want any special treatment. When Sarah went into labour, the hospital started behaving in a way that we now know was going to end to disaster. In the early hours of the morning the midwife said she couldn't find our baby's heartbeat. A doctor explained that it was because Sarah's bladder was full, but when they drained it they just said, 'I'm sorry, your baby's dead' and walked out. Our world fell apart.

When Harriet died, Sarah and I tried to carry on, but there was an extraordinary numbness; we just existed. We couldn't bring ourselves to even drive past the hospital any more, so we moved out to a little village in the Peak District.

We kept Harriet's beautiful, poor little body in their freezer for nearly two years because we didn't want to do something final. It's horrible to say but we didn't want to dispose of the evidence – that's the reality. All the way through, the hospital kept denying our account of what had happened. We know now there had been serious safety issues for years and it was clear that more babies would die if we didn't say anything. We had to challenge them, but it was so difficult after what we had been through.

We'd go on walks together in the Peaks or up to the Yorkshire Dales, and I would spend two or three hours staring at Sarah's heels as she walked, not able to look up.

Not being allowed to grieve – or being actively prevented from grieving – made it even worse. The hospital was our employer, but we had no help, no occupational input and no support whatsoever from them. We were just left alone. What's more, we both lost our jobs.

Sometimes it felt like we didn't even have each other any more. Our relationship was under huge strain, as we were grieving differently and at different times. Often, I think I showed sadness as anger, so instead of saying, 'I'm sad and need a hug' I would shout.

JOURNEY TO RECOVERY

I've had different types of therapy, including EMDR and CBT, but it wasn't until five years after Harriet died that I started grief counselling. It was deeply emotional and helped me. We spent a long time fighting to get an independent review into maternity services at the hospital, and now I feel an enormous sense of relief at no longer having to fight that battle. It has given me a different way of living; I can be more vulnerable, and I cry much more easily.

NOT FORGETTING

Now we have another daughter, Lottie. Often when people see me with her they ask whether I have any more children. I say, 'Yes, I've got two' and if they ask about our second child I tell them that they're not alive. It's the truth. I'm never going to pretend. I'm always going to be Harriet's dad. What I think is really important about my journey is that I can help Lottie to understand that grief is normal and that the way to deal with it is to be honest and ask for help. My grief recovery work was amazing. It showed me that big boys can cry; they don't have to be tough.

FUTURE DEVELOPMENTS

PREDICTING VULNERABILITY TO TRAUMA

While we think of trauma as being unanticipated and personal, we can in some circumstances predict where people are likely to develop PTSD. At a societal level, wars and natural disasters can cause a surge in cases of PTSD, while on an individual level events such as difficult childbirth or the death of a family member are known to trigger the condition. People in certain professions also tend to be exposed to traumatic events, such as those in the emergency services, military, police and social services.

Several different approaches are proving successful in either preventing PTSD or limiting its severity if it does develop. These include identifying those who potentially may be at greater risk of developing PTSD and building up resilience by enabling a shift in thinking patterns so they can frame trauma differently. This has been used with those working in emergency services and with paramedic students, in projects such as SHAPE, discussed above.

ACCESSIBILITY AND SCALABILITY OF TREATMENTS

When trauma occurs at a large scale, for example due to a pandemic, natural disaster or national conflict, PTSD treatments need to be simple to administer outside traditional professional settings and by non-specialists. They need to be accessible, scalable and able to be administered as soon as possible after the event to prevent PTSD setting in or worsening.

One treatment that is proving to be effective as a means of early intervention involves the individual engaging in a task or game to try to disrupt the usual mechanism by which intrusive memories are recalled and laid down. This approach can be used

'There are very few predictors of what makes people more resilient to trauma than others and trying to identify individual variables isn't the most helpful approach. The strongest predictor of PTSD is how many previous repeated episodes of trauma have been experienced. Because of this, I believe we have dose-wise response to trauma as we can with a virus. And, like a virus, I believe we can one day have interventions, similar to vaccinations, that can protect us if they are put in place as soon after the trauma as possible.'

PROFESSOR EMILY HOLMES

as early as six hours after the trauma. Researchers (including Dr Emily Holmes, as we saw earlier) have described these approaches as 'vaccines', as they can protect people from developing PTSD by working on a mechanism that is central to its development. The challenge now is to develop larger-scale trials and with different groups of people.

DIVERSITY AND SPECTRUM OF TRAUMA

While in many people's minds PTSD is linked to the experience of former military veterans, it can affect anyone. Indeed, many more people may be experiencing some form of PTSD than have been diagnosed. More research is needed to explore the behaviours that might enable people to cope with, but also hide, their PTSD, thereby preventing recovery. In cases of complex PTSD, these coping mechanisms may be very entrenched as a result of years of ongoing trauma. Linked to this is a need for more research into possible indications of PTSD that may be more subtle and difficult to detect.

Ultimately, researchers hope that by discovering more about the mechanisms behind PTSD, whether they be genetic, biological or within our thought processes, they will be able to develop more effective treatments.

'Trauma doesn't just set into motion PTSD, it sets into motion all sorts of conditions that can build up. So if we need to reach a lot of people we want simple tools, based in scientific research, that don't need professionals to deliver them so we can scale them up. My dream would be that we could use science to develop these approaches and then it could go straight into the hands of people who can deliver them quickly and at scale.'

PROFESSOR EMILY HOLMES

SPOTLIGHT ON BIG DATA: UNCOVERING PATTERNS AND EMPOWERING VOICES IN MENTAL HEALTH

POWER OF BIG DATA AND DATA LINKAGE

Researchers are using routinely collected data to investigate trends in mental health and their connections to other factors. Routinely collected anonymous data is sourced from NHS electronic health records, the National Pupil Database, social service records, legal/judicial records and census information. The data from these different sources can then be linked to build a bigger picture of our mental health by nesting it within the context of social, environmental, genetic, educational and other factors.

There are many advantages to working with data in this way. Firstly, the large numbers give statistical power to the analysis so findings are more robust than research using smaller samples. They also speak clearly to policymakers because of the numbers involved. Secondly, the data is generated in real life so people are not excluded or missed. Traditional research or clinical trials select a group of people to study and try to control for variables that may influence findings as a means to show that something does work and there isn't another explanation. Routine data doesn't do this, which makes the data messier but more real.

The datasets follow people anonymously over time so it is possible to look at trajectories and observe transitions.

Lastly, applying big data approaches brings different specialists together. Not only does this paint a more holistic picture but it also allows people to question the language they use in their own specialisms and the assumptions they make in research.

'When I think about mental health, I think about diagnosis, function, and impairment and context, and it's the interaction of all those things that actually tells you how a person will be experiencing their problem. So I think yes, big data will take us down the path of having much more tailored interventions for people with mental health problems, but I think it will equally take us down the path of actually, in certain circumstances that diagnosis doesn't matter.'

PROFESSOR ANN JOHN

FINDING HIDDEN PATTERNS BUT NOT ALWAYS EXPLANATIONS

Routinely collected data allows researchers to examine who gets referred to which services, but it also enables assessment of who gets seen in terms of attending their first, second, third or fourth appointment. This allows researchers to identify where and when people fall through the net, identifying inequalities among groups in terms of access and engagement.

It can also uncover patterns that would not necessarily be visible. For example, if young people who are under 16 present to an emergency department with self-harm the official guidance is that they should be admitted overnight for assessment. This doesn't always happen, and analysis of data on hospital admissions has shown that girls are much more likely to be admitted than boys.[15] This is regardless of what method of self-harm was used, whether that be overdose or cutting. This finding raises the question of whether this trend is because we view self-harm differently in girls and boys or because we respond to boys and girls in distress differently. Similarly, recent research has shown that those with English as a second language are less likely to be seen at hospital for self-harm.[16] This may not be because there is less self-harm in this group but because of variations in help-seeking behaviour. In both cases big data analysis has been able to uncover these patterns but not provide explanations; this may require further surveys or interview research.

REFRAMING PROBLEMS AS RISK FACTORS

Research in the *Lancet Psychiatry* linked data from schools on absences and exclusion with GP and hospital data for all young people up to the age of 24 who had a mental health diagnosis. The research showed that a diagnosis of some mental health conditions was 6–7 times higher in those young people with higher absences or exclusion from school.[17]

Our educational system tends to focus on 100 per cent attendance, but what this analysis is indicating is that young people who are getting excluded or who aren't coming to school have a high level of mental health problems. This means we could use this routinely collected data on absence/exclusion to identify young people who are in need of extra support. Although this isn't a surprise, it is a clear demonstration in the data that this is the case.

So rather than being just an indicator of a successful school or individual attainment, absence/exclusion is also an indicator that a young person needs support, and identifying the young people who need support to prevent those poor outcomes involves a much more complex picture.

WHERE NOW?

If you, or a loved one, has experienced a traumatic event then it is normal to have upsetting and confusing thoughts and feelings afterwards. For most people, these improve over a few weeks and talking to friends and family is always helpful.

If you or a child are still having problems four weeks after a traumatic incident, or if your symptoms are particularly troublesome (such as experiencing flashbacks or not being able to sleep), then you should reach out to your GP in the first instance.

Remember, it doesn't matter how long ago the experience was, nor how you or anyone else perceives its severity. Everyone reacts differently to trauma; however, the right support can help everyone, and PTSD can be effectively treated at any time, even years after the initial event.

Your GP will need to carry out a detailed assessment of your symptoms as there are many different ways to treat PTSD and they will need to determine the best one for you. They might refer you to a specialist to carry out this assessment, and in some cases you can refer yourself to a psychological therapy service.

Sometimes, and particularly if the traumatic incident happened recently, your doctor might ask you to record your symptoms for a period of time to see if they change. This is called active monitoring and it helps your doctor to make a more accurate diagnosis and determine the best course of action.

In most cases of PTSD, psychological therapies are recommended, such as talking therapies or group therapy sessions.

There are different psychological therapies used in the treatment of PTSD:

COGNITIVE BEHAVIOURAL THERAPY (CBT) OR TRAUMA FOCUSED COGNITIVE BEHAVIOURAL THERAPY (TF-CBT)

This is a type of talking therapy aimed to help you manage symptoms by changing thinking processes and the way you act. CBT sessions are usually between 60 and 90 minutes long and are delivered weekly for a period of 8 to 12 weeks.

EYE MOVEMENT DESENSITISATION AND REPROCESSING (EMDR)

EMDR is a type of therapy that involves recalling the traumatic incident in detail while making specific eye movements such as following your therapist's finger.

Your doctor might also advise a course of medication depending on your symptoms. A particular type of antidepressant called selective serotonin reuptake inhibitors or SSRIs have been shown to be effective in treating symptoms of complex PTSD in some people.

When it comes to treating PTSD, there are different approaches and you shouldn't be disheartened if you find that what your doctor first recommends hasn't improved your symptoms after 8 to 10 weeks. Instead, you should let your doctor know that you have not seen an improvement so that they can either recommend a different approach or refer you to a specialist.

If you are not ready to speak to your doctor, or if you are worried about someone else, then there are a number of charities offering advice and support:

Mind.org.uk

Mind offers advice, legal information and support both on their website and over the phone. Their helpline is open 365 days a year from 6pm to 11pm on 0300 123 3393.

For victims of crime or violence:

VictimSupport.org.uk

Victim Support offer free and confidential advice 24/7 on 0808 1689111, or you can use their web chat service.

RapeCrisis.org.uk

Rape Crisis are working to end sexual assault and offer support to victims over the age of 16, no matter how severe or long ago an incident occurred. You can call them on 0808 500 2222 24/7 or use their online chat function through the website.

For children and young people:

Childline.org.uk

Childline offer support and advice to children and young people on a range of topics. They can be contacted 24/7 on 0800 1111. They also offer an online web chat service.

For military veterans:

PTSDresolution.org

PTSD Resolution offer counselling services for force veterans and reservists. They can be contacted during office hours on 0300 302 0551

For new parents:

BirthTraumaAssociation.org.uk

The Birth Trauma Association offer peer to peer support over email via support@birthtraumaassociation.org.uk

For more information about MQ's work into PTSD, and the latest research findings, visit:

the experts

EMILY HOLMES

Emily Holmes leads the Emotional Mental Imagery Lab (EMIL) at Uppsala University. Her research is underpinned by a core interest in mental health science, and the translation of basic findings to create innovations to improve psychological treatments. She studied psychology and philosophy at university before going to art college. When she lived in New York she did voluntary work with homeless people and it was during this time she realised that psychological ill health played an important role in where we end up in life. She decided to train to become a clinical psychologist in the UK and her first job was in a traumatic stress clinic in central London. With a continuing interest in the visual aspect of psychology, she was compelled to understand the flashbacks and intrusive memories that are so integral to PTSD. She enrolled to do a PhD to investigate the fundamental question of why mental images have a more powerful impact on our emotions than verbal thoughts. As she studied she continued to work clinically, keeping her research grounded in the lived experience of her patients. When she finished her PhD she continued researching mental imagery, looking at flash-forwards as well as flashbacks and developing ways to study the mechanisms involved in imagery. She continues to work at the boundary of research and clinical work.

PROFESSOR JENNIFER WILD

Professor Jennifer Wild is a consultant clinical psychologist and professor of military mental health at the University of Melbourne with affiliate status at the University of Oxford. Her area of expertise is in developing and evaluating evidence-based interventions for improving resilience to stress, including PTSD and complex grief. From a young age she was interested in psychology and when she studied the subject at university she soon became fascinated with memory. In particular she was interested in the role of memory in PTSD and, in her doctorate, she studied how the brain creates a memory and then rewrites it after therapy. After her doctorate she specialised in researching people who are regularly exposed to traumatic events, such as emergency service workers, military personnel and journalists working in conflict zones. She also became dedicated to raising awareness of common disorders and their effective treatment. She is enthusiastic about communicating science and regularly contributes articles to the press about trauma-related problems and appears in the media giving expert commentary on psychological issues.

For Ann John's bio please see Chapter 5.

4

eating disorders

INTRODUCTION

Eating disorders form a complex set of mental health conditions that revolve around our relationship with food, eating, weight and body image. They are influenced by a myriad of factors, ranging from our genes to the values embedded in our culture and society. They can have a devastating impact. Anorexia nervosa has been shown to have the highest mortality rate of any mental health condition. Bulimia and binge eating, meanwhile, are associated with severe medical complications, such as kidney failure, heart problems, gastrointestinal damage, tooth decay and gum disease. In every case, an eating disorder will severely affect the life of the sufferer and the people who care for them.

It is estimated that around 1.25 million people in the UK have an eating disorder,[1] although more research is needed to determine how widespread these conditions are. Eating disorders are often kept hidden because, as with other mental health conditions, there is often a lot of accompanying shame. For many, eating disorders are a coping mechanism to deal with difficult emotions and experiences. The person may fear that speaking out about their condition will mean having to give up a habit that they consider helpful or even essential, and to which they feel they have no alternative.

'It wasn't a lifestyle choice. Perhaps it wasn't really a choice at all. It was a solution that presented itself to me when I didn't really have any others, and I really needed help.'

JAMES DOWNS

Due to media coverage, awareness around the impact of eating disorders is growing, but it has failed to convey the diversity of those affected by these conditions. For example, around 25 per cent of those affected by an eating disorder are male and, although eating disorders often start in young people aged 13 to 17, recent research shows that up to 6.4 per cent of adults display signs of having one. Stories and imagery around eating disorders tend also to feature white, middle-class teenagers, although they actually affect people from ethnically and socioeconomically diverse backgrounds.

Eating disorders are long-lasting conditions and they are becoming increasingly common. Between April and December 2021 almost 10,000 children and young people started treatment for an eating disorder. This was reflected in a record demand for services, up one-quarter compared to the same period in 2020 and by almost two-thirds since before the pandemic.[2]

An eating disorder diagnosis is based on an assessment of eating patterns, but includes checks on weight, blood samples and BMI. While its medical definition has a very physical basis, there are many psychological and social layers that also need to be considered when developing and implementing treatments.

'Over my lifetime anorexia has moved from mainstream health into psychiatry but there is still a problem around where we belong and some of us that work in this area feel that we have never really been accepted. Now genetic research is showing that eating disorders are rather different to the rest of psychiatry as they also have this metabolic link. Anorexia is linked to low BMI and insulin sensitivity (whereas the binge spectrum disorders have the opposite profile, i.e. links with higher BMI and insulin resistance). Thus eating disorders fit the profile of a psychosomatic illness, with physical profiles interacting with mental factors at a critical phase of development within a particular environment .'

PROFESSOR JANET TREASURE

COMPLEXITY OF EATING DISORDERS

Our relationship with food has become complex. At a societal level, food has come to symbolise more than simply nutrition; it is part of our culture. Society also presents us with expectations about what our bodies should look like and what is considered attractive.

At an individual level, food is one of the many mediums through which our emotions and distress can be expressed. This is established early in life when we first start to feed, but emotional attachments with food may develop throughout our lifetimes, depending on our genes, metabolic make-up, family upbringing, peers and culture.

Eating disorders have become increasingly widespread over the years. The reasons for this are difficult to ascertain but may, in part, be due to greater awareness and recognition. Eating disorders were previously confined to the outskirts of medical care, treated as a physical health condition, with a focus on the impact of food restriction on the body. The medical definition of an eating disorder that relies on BMI is to some extent a legacy of this.

As more research was conducted into eating disorders, they moved under the umbrella of mental health conditions and into the realms of psychiatry and psychology. As 'in-between' conditions that still remain somewhat hidden by society, eating disorders require more recognition and more support for associated research and services. It is estimated that eating disorders cost the UK £8.8 billion in 2019 and £9.4 billion in 2020, yet they remain underfunded.[3]

DIFFERENT FORMS

Currently, there are considered to be three main eating disorders: anorexia nervosa, bulimia and binge-eating disorder. People can develop just one of these conditions or they can move between them. Exact prevalence rates of these eating disorders are difficult to gauge. A 2017 study in Australia[4] showed that anorexia accounted for 8 per cent of cases, avoidant/restrictive food intake disorder (ARFID) 5 per cent, binge-eating disorder 22 per cent, bulimia 19 per cent, and other specified feeding or eating disorder (OSFED) 47 per cent.

People with **anorexia** (anorexia nervosa) develop a low weight by limiting how much they eat and drink. They may develop 'rules' around what they can and cannot eat, as well as when and where. Alongside this, they may exercise excessively, make themselves sick or misuse laxatives. Some people with anorexia may experience cycles of bingeing (eating large amounts of food at once) and then purging.

People with **bulimia** are caught in a cycle of eating large quantities of food and then trying to compensate by vomiting, taking laxatives or diuretics, fasting or exercising excessively (purging).

People with **binge-eating disorder** (BED) eat large quantities of food over a short period of time. Unlike people with bulimia, they don't usually follow this by getting rid of the food, but may fast between binges. BED is not about choosing to eat large portions for enjoyment. In fact, binges tend to be very distressing, often involving a much larger amount of food than someone would want to eat. Characteristics of a binge-eating episode can include eating much faster than normal, eating until feeling uncomfortably full, eating large amounts of food when not physically hungry, eating alone through embarrassment at the amount being eaten, and feelings of disgust, shame or guilt during or after the binge.

THE PHYSICAL IMPACT

Anorexia can cause severe physical problems because of the effects of starvation on the body. It can lead to loss of both muscle and bone strength, and women and girls whose periods have previously started may find that they stop. They may also find that their sex drive decreases, which can have different impacts on males and females.

Bulimia can also cause serious physical complications. Frequent vomiting can cause problems with the teeth, and harm may be caused to the individual by the process of making themselves sick. Laxative misuse, meanwhile, can seriously affect the heart and digestive system.

There are many ways that binge-eating disorder can impact on a person's life. Often, though not always, it causes weight gain, and in terms of physical health is associated with high blood pressure, high cholesterol, type 2 diabetes and heart disease.

EMOTIONAL DRIVERS

Weight and shape tend to play a large role in how much self-worth someone with anorexia feels. The way they view themselves is often at odds with how others see them, so they have a distorted image of themselves and think that they're larger than they really are (see the section on body image and brain changes, p.194). They experience a deep fear of gaining weight and will usually challenge the idea that they should do so.

Binge eating is often a way to cope with difficult emotions; someone may feel driven to binge eat if they're feeling stressed, upset or angry, for example. While bingeing, people with bulimia don't feel in control of how much or how quickly they're eating, and the food eaten during a binge may include things the person would usually avoid. People with bulimia place strong emphasis on their weight and shape, and may see themselves as much larger than they really are. Some people with bulimia or BED have described feeling disconnected from what they're doing during a binge, and even struggle to remember what they've eaten afterwards.

Difficult or overwhelming feelings, such as feeling low, bored, angry, upset or anxious, can make someone feel the urge to binge eat. However, people may also binge eat when they are feeling happy or excited. Sometimes binge-eating episodes may even be more habitual or planned, rather than driven by a sudden urge. There are a number of reasons for this, including feeling numb or unable to manage uncomfortable feelings.

CAUSES OF EATING DISORDERS

Many people with lived experience of an eating disorder cannot pinpoint a single event or experience as its cause. Most health professionals believe that there is a combination of factors that lead to the development of an eating disorder; it is likely to be influenced by a build-up of emotions and experiences, rather than a single trigger.

Identifying these risk factors may prove useful in helping to predict someone's susceptibility to developing an eating disorder. However, given the typically long-lasting nature of these conditions, it's also important to examine the factors that maintain them.

Based on what we know about the metabolic and genetic patterns of the different eating disorders, theories have developed around their distinct genetic basis and evolutionary function. One of these is that the triggering event is a change in eating patterns, whether that be starvation, bingeing, a conscious diet or restriction of food due to illness. In the modern world there may be many reasons for such a change in diet, but they would once have been linked only to the availability of food. It has been suggested that when an anorexic limits their food intake it triggers high physical activity, as we have self-regulating mechanisms aimed at enabling us to search for food in times of famine.[5]

For those who develop binge eating, one theory is that eating food when it's available, despite satiety, is a necessary trait in environments where an intensive supply of food may be followed by long stretches with none. It may be a survival advantage to have a genetic make-up that enables you to eat more during the times when food is available.[6] Research suggests that people with low BMI and insulin sensitivity may be more prone to anorexia, while those with higher BMI and insulin resistance may be more likely to develop bulimia and binge-eating disorders.

Other evolutionary theories for eating disorders relate to sexual selection and the suppression of reproduction in the context of food availability. It is possible that a combination of these different evolutionary explanations is the genetic basis of eating disorders. Large-scale research projects, such as the Eating Disorders Genetics Initiative (EDGI)[7] aim to better understand the role of our genes and environment in the development of eating disorders. EDGI in the UK collects psychological, medical and genetic information from 10,000 people with experience of eating disorders; it is part of an international collaboration, with many countries coming together as part of the same initiative. The end goal is that, by understanding these conditions better, healthcare might become better equipped to support and treat those people experiencing them.

'In some ways the conditions that fall within eating disorders differ and in some ways they are the same. Research is indicating they have different profiles in terms of the other mental health conditions that accompany them, so anorexia is associated with obsessive compulsive disorder and autism spectrum disorder. Possibly some of the underlying mechanisms in the body and the brain are the same but skewed in different ways depending on whether people constantly restrict their eating or go through stages of bingeing. I think now we're beginning to see that there are variations and the options to personalise treatment and formulate each one rather differently.'

PROFESSOR JANET TREASURE

SIGNS AND SYMPTOMS

Anorexia Nervosa:

Food fixation: constantly thinking about food, counting calories

Low self-esteem: constantly feeling you are never good enough

Food avoidance: due to a need for control, reducing food intake

Secretive: hiding food or lying about how much you have eaten

Anxious: increase in anxiety around mealtimes

Bulimia Nervosa:

A repeated cycle: binge eating or eating large amounts of food in a short period of time, then purging

Loss of control: over how much you eat, then feeling ashamed for overcompensating

Low self-esteem: based on body shape and weight

Binge-eating disorder:

Low self-esteem: emptiness, shame or feeling that you're never good enough

Poor self-regulation: you can't stop eating and may eat large amounts all at once

Comfort eating: eating as a coping mechanism

Secretive: hiding, or lying about, how much you have eaten

Weight gain: as a result of binge eating

Poor health: including breathlessness and fatigue

SCOFF QUESTIONNAIRE

This screening tool was developed as a way to flag up possible eating disorders. A score of two or more positive answers is a positive result. Questions include:

Do you ever make yourself **s**ick because you feel uncomfortably full?

Do you worry you have lost **c**ontrol over how much you eat?

Have you recently lost more than **o**ne stone (6 kilos) over a three-month period?

Do you believe yourself to be **f**at when others say you are too thin?

Would you say that **f**ood dominates your life?

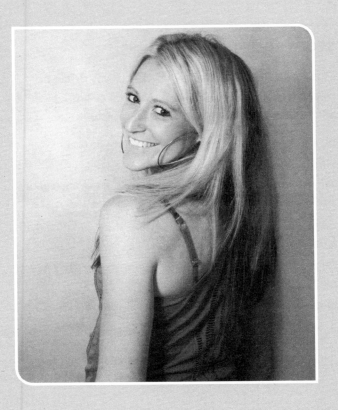

Hope Virgo is an advocate and campaigner for people with eating disorders and founded the #DumpTheScales campaign, which calls on the UK government to review the guidance relating to eating disorders. She is the author of three books, Stand Tall Little Girl, Hope Through Recovery and the most recent You Are Free (Even If You Don't Feel Like It).

I developed anorexia when I was about 12 or 13 and I'm still in ongoing recovery in my thirties. I was sexually abused at around the same age, but although I'm sure that contributed to my eating disorder I don't think that it was the only factor. I always struggled with emotions and I felt that there was something categorically wrong with me. Restricting my food intake and obsessively exercising became a way for me to get rid of these emotions

VOICE IN MY HEAD

I often think about anorexia as a voice in my head or a bad friend. One that would tell me on a day-to-day basis what to eat, what to drink and how much exercise I should be doing. The more I listened to what the voice was telling me the better I felt about everything else. It numbed all those emotions and it helped me feel maybe I was good enough and things would work out. It felt like it was helping me and I hid it from my family and friends for about four years. It was when my school got in touch with my mum about their concerns that I went to CAMHS.

Even when I had been referred I remained in the grips of anorexia. I didn't want to accept there was anything the matter with me and whenever anyone tried to talk to me I would shut down and pretend I was fine. But slowly I began to realise that I was really unhappy. Most evenings I would sit with all of these emotions and intense feelings of guilt. On those evenings I would wish something would click in my brain so I could be like everybody else. I'd make this promise to change, but then I'd get up in the morning and weigh myself, look in the mirror and nothing would have shifted. My brain just wouldn't let me make those changes. Eventually I got admitted to hospital.

For me thinking of anorexia as a voice helps because I can distance myself from it. When I was in treatment and since leaving I sometimes write letters to the eating disorder because it helps me vocalise how bad I think it is and how it's trying to ruin things for me.

LONG ROAD TO RECOVERY

One of the key moments for me in my recovery was realising my body image was so distorted. On my third day in hospital one of the nurses made me draw a life-size version of what I thought I looked like, and then she traced around my own body – it made me see my body image was completely different to reality. That helped me to trust the staff in the hospital and to start thinking maybe I could change. Then the more I began to live my life and get that freedom and the spontaneity back, the more I saw how much the eating disorder had limited my social activity and everything that I wanted to do.

But even when I was recovering the voice would come back and use my feelings as a chance to pull me back in. It often romanticised how anorexia made me feel and made me think it was so much better when I wasn't eating. This made me forget all the negatives of living with an eating disorder: the lack of energy and the constant obsession with food.

Ever since discharge I've been in an ongoing state of recovery. When I left hospital I was very institutionalised – I didn't know how to eat or what to do on a day-to-day basis. So I stuck to the meal plans but looking back I don't know how much my thinking had actually changed. I relapsed in 2016 and now I am trying to work really hard to do that final shift in my thinking and thought processes.

For me therapy helps, especially during my recent pregnancy, but I think what has been most useful is proactively challenging my thinking about food and my fear of foods, making sure that I'm communicating in the right way and knowing that if I keep pushing things will slowly slot more into place.

IT'S NOT ABOUT THE FOOD

Anorexia gave me what I thought was control, but I've realised that actually it gave me a sense of certainty. A certainty that the fear was going to be managed and I wasn't going to feel. That's why I go to these behaviours because they numb the emotion and give me certainty that it will go away, that everything will be fine. But actually in reality it makes things much worse – it never delivers on what it's promising you.

For me eating disorders aren't really about the food or the exercise or my body image. What I've learnt is that for me it's about the fear and not being able to communicate and needing to stifle these feelings. When I'm really stressed or anxious or unhappy I project all of those feelings onto my body and then the eating disorder uses that to pull me back in. Now I'm better at being able to predict that my brain's going to respond like that, so I can use mantras and various coping mechanisms to stop me going down the path of eating disorders.

SOCIETY AND MEDIA

I think that our society has got this embedded eating disorder culture where everyone's talking about their bodies, food and dieting and constantly trying to change themselves to feel good enough.

Most people don't really understand EDs and see them as a choice or a phase people go through. People don't understand that it is a mental health issue and I think part of this is because it has this very physical element behind it, which makes it much more complex. The media also portrays it as a white middle-class teenage girl's illness when actually we know they present in all different body sizes, and I think because of that we see that stigma not only in society but across healthcare and the government. And this is why we don't get enough funding, which creates this vicious cycle as it's just not given the support it needs.

PHYSICAL AND MENTAL

I don't agree with using BMI as a measure of whether someone has anorexia and needs services. It can lead to people being excluded from the support they need and it means people don't get the right space to really listen to their body and fully understand what they need. When I came out of hospital I stuck religiously to my meal plan because I knew that then my BMI would stay exactly the same and this would give me this sense of security and certainty that actually maintained my eating disorders.

When you're in recovery you need to have a multidisciplinary team around you, so that you understand all the different factors and see how it's all intertwined. At the moment we tend to consider it as needing a basic treatment around food intake so people get to a healthy weight and are discharged and then they're very likely to relapse or never make that full recovery.

ROLE OF RESEARCH

I think people look for a cause for their eating disorder because they want answers and they want to have someone or something to blame. I think that research can help people to understand that EDs are much more complicated than many of us think and, alongside helping people recover, this can shift the blame and the thinking around it.

I'd like research to give us a better understanding about the brain chemistry: how that links to people developing eating disorders and how that keeps people stuck when they're in that recovery space. And I think we need to examine more closely what treatments do and don't work for different people: I don't think you can have a one size fits all when it comes to treatment.

INTERNAL MAINTENANCE OF THE CONDITION

BRAIN CHANGES

Research has shown that eating disorders can affect the brain in a number of ways, and that these changes may play a role in the continuation of symptoms. The brains of people who have, or have had, anorexia differ subtly in their structure and chemical pathways compared to those of people who have had no experience of the disorder. These differences are thought to play a role in how people with eating disorders respond to, and manage, rewards. Given that food is one of our most basic rewards, it would make sense if it were involved in the development and maintenance of eating disorders.

Further investigations are underway to better understand the brain's response to feedback and reward. Recent research on the brain scans of 2,000 people with anorexia,[8] for example, showed 'sizeable reductions' in three critical measures of brain structure: the thickness and surface area of the cortex (the outer layer of the brain), and the volume of brain structures that sit directly beneath the cortex. It is thought that a reduction in brain size implies a loss of brain cells or the connections between them. When the researchers compared their findings with similar studies on other conditions, they found that brain changes in anorexia were some two to four times greater than in conditions such as depression, ADHD or OCD. The researchers found that reductions in brain structure were less severe, meanwhile, among people in recovery from anorexia. This suggests that the changes are not permanent and that, with appropriate treatment and support, the brain may be able to repair itself.

'It's not so much the trigger that's important, but the maintaining factors that suck people in and trap them. Once someone has anorexia it tends to persist for a long time – on average seven years – so it's very unlike other psychiatric disorders, which sort of wax and wane. It's persistent, and it tends to start at a key time in development, so a lot of milestones are put on hold.'

PROFESSOR JANET TREASURE

REWARD CIRCUITRY

Individuals with anorexia tend to have more difficulty experiencing pleasure than non-anorexics, and can more easily refrain from experiences that would be considered to be fun or enjoyable. They find it difficult to enjoy a reward or the anticipation of it, in part because of concerns over the consequences[9] and what might happen to their body if they eat. They also often think that everything they do is wrong or flawed and have a high sensitivity to criticism. Even faced with the praise or belief of others, people with eating disorders find it difficult to proportion reward and punishment appropriately.

Imaging data has shown that the brains of people who have, or have had, anorexia have an underactive limbic circuity, part of the brain that relates to feelings of reward. They also have more active executive circuits in the brain; these relate to the planning and inhibition of actions in consideration of future consequences.

The brains of people with anorexia also have a persistent disturbance in their serotonin chemical pathways, which may be linked to increased anxiety.[10] It is unknown whether this anxiety is caused by, or contributes to, the anorexia.

Research has shown that the brains of people with eating disorders respond differently to food or pictures of food. Imaging studies,[11] where people's brains are scanned while they are asked to think about eating the food depicted, have shown that women with anorexia and bulimia activate more top-down control centres in the brain in response to food images. Women with bulimia have increased activation in the reward regions of the brain as well as increased activation in the control centres, which may play off against each other.

This suggests that people with bulimia have an increased response in terms of their appetite and action when they see or experience food. In parallel, they have varying (and perhaps sporadic) levels of inhibition in the area of the brain responsible for attention and planning. This may explain why they tend to yo-yo between bingeing and purging. Those with anorexia, in comparison, show an increased inhibition of thought processes in response to seeing food, but not an increased activation in the reward areas of the brain.

Researchers have also looked at the notion of reward using a well-known guessing game where participants try to win or lose money. People recovering from anorexia[12] were compared to those who had no experience of an eating disorder. Results showed that the healthy group responded with very different

Bulimic > Anorexic patients

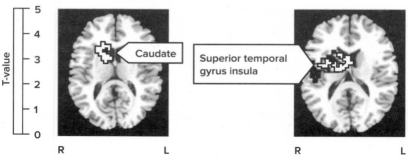

BETWEEN-GROUP MAP ACTIVATION SHOWING FOOD/NON-FOOD ACTIVATION IN
WOMEN WITH BULIMIA NERVOSA VERSUS ANOREXIA NERVOSA

neural brain activity when they won money than when they lost it. The people who had recovered from anorexia, however, had similar brain reactions to both winning and losing. These results suggest that people with anorexia may have trouble distinguishing between positive and negative feedback. This could help to explain why it is difficult to motivate anorexia patients in treatment or convince them of the consequences of their behaviours.

Researchers have also used imaging to study brain responses during a taste-reward task, where women received or were denied an unexpected sweet stimulus (sugar solution).[13] Those with eating disorders, higher BMI and binge-eating behaviours showed less surprise at this 'reward' than those without eating disorders. These women also showed very different brain activation during this task in areas connected to reward. These results suggest that, for women with eating disorders, the normal response to reward has been altered, meaning they are able to override hunger cues. In contrast, the opposite seems to be the case for women with binge-eating episodes and higher BMIs.

CAN WE PREDICT AN EATING DISORDER FROM BRAIN IMAGING?

Research as part of the IMAGEN project[14] analysed data from 1,386 healthy adolescents from eight countries. Using brain scans and measures of depression, anxiety, attention deficit hyperactivity disorder (ADHD), conduct disorder and emotional problems, the study compared adolescents who did and didn't develop three types of disordered eating behaviours (dieting, binge eating and purging) over a period of five years. The presence of these behaviours did not necessarily mean that the young people had eating disorders, but indicated their eating was different from most. Analysis showed that all three types of disordered eating behaviours developed alongside signs of depression, whereas signs of ADHD and conduct disorder pre-dated the development of unhealthy eating behaviours.

Adolescents who developed both disordered eating behaviours and depressive symptoms showed differences in volume in certain brain areas at the age of 14. More specifically, the study showed that the development of binge-eating behaviours was predicted at the age of 14 by larger volumes of grey matter in parts of the striatum, an area usually involved in reward processing. In contrast, the development of both purging behaviours and signs of depression was predicted by lower volumes of grey matter in areas of the prefrontal cortex, which is associated with control and decision-making. This aligns with findings of brain differences in people who have been diagnosed with anorexia or binge-eating disorder.

THOUGHT PROCESSES

People with eating disorders think and process information in quite distinct ways, but their patterns and qualities of thinking have similarities with other mental health conditions. The preoccupation with food and weight in eating disorders has parallels with what is observed in anxiety and OCD, where there is a tendency to ruminate and dwell on certain subjects. Similarly, people with depression typically display an all-or-nothing way of thinking and catastrophise when something negative, but relatively small, has happened. Alongside this, the ability of people with eating disorders to completely focus on certain behaviours and their difficulty with social interactions has been compared to how people with autism think. There is also thought to be an element of addictive behaviour observed in people with eating disorders.

There is continuing debate about whether these thinking patterns pre-date the onset of eating disorders, or if they are caused by the condition over the years. There is also uncertainty around the longevity of the impact of eating disorders on thinking. Some propose that if changes in thinking are the result of malnourishment, then thought processes should return to normal after recovery. Others believe that differences in thinking continue even when brain is being nourished again. It is unlikely that we will find definitive answers to these debates, as it will depend in part on how thought processes are measured[15] and vary from one individual to another.

BODY IMAGE

Body image disturbance (BID), where an individual experiences his or her shape or weight differently from how it is in reality, is a key part of eating disorders.[16] According to research, BID has two key components, the first being a perceptual difficulty

'People with eating disorders can be more rigid in their thinking and less able to see the bigger picture. All of these cognitive, emotional and social changes mean that people can get stuck in a pattern of behaviour, and there is a growing interest in the link with autism. However, we can't be sure if these behaviours and thinking patterns are there before eating disorders develop or are a result of these conditions. Currently it seems that perhaps there's 5 per cent of people who have autism early on and then go on to develop eating disorders, but more generally research tells us that people with eating disorders consistently experience difficulties with aspects of social and emotional behaviour, which impacts their relationships. It seems that these difficulties are made worse by starvation and do improve in recovery.'

PROFESSOR JANET TREASURE

estimating one's own body size and dimensions (typically judged to be bigger than in reality). The second component is to do with the person's thinking patterns around social judgements, and is commonly displayed in very negative attitudes and emotions towards their own body.

Despite the key role of BID in predicting the onset, treatment outcome and future relapse of eating disorders, there has been some debate about how insight around this might influence treatment and support. Attempts to challenge someone's perception of their body are likely to be met with hostility and refusal, but it may be possible to work with their more general attitudes about what is considered overweight. Recent studies suggest that BID can be reduced using a form of training that works with our biases around weight and body. This approach does not attempt to change a person's judgements about their own body size directly, but instead focuses on how they categorise a body of a particular size. It aims to recalibrate the boundary at which bodies are judged to be overweight. This challenges the person's preconceptions about what constitutes an acceptable body size, enabling them to have a more accurate sense of their own body.

This approach is called cognitive bias training and uses computer-generated imagery (CGI) to show a continuum of body sizes, from emaciated to obese.[17] The patient is asked to locate the point along the continuum that represents their subjective judgement of the transition from a 'thin' to a 'fat' body (i.e. the categorical boundary). The training procedure then aims to shift this boundary towards heavier bodies (see the figures opposite).

Research shows that this training is effective at enabling this shift and is accompanied by a significant reduction in the participants' concerns about their own body shape and weight, and eating. One month later, the progress made by patients was found to have been retained.

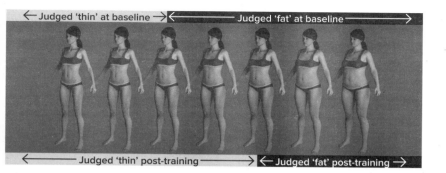

IMAGES USED IN A STUDY EVALUATING COGNITIVE BIAS TRAINING AS A MEANS TO ADDRESS BDI

EXTERNAL MAINTENANCE

TREATMENT FOR ADULTS

Cognitive behavioural therapy – During CBT, a therapist will try to help the patient cope with their feelings, understand the importance of nutrition and the effects of starvation, and make healthy food choices. They will ask that the patient practises these techniques on their own and then measures their progress.

Specialist supportive clinical management – SSCM involves talking to a therapist to help understand the causes of the eating disorder, as well as to discuss nutrition and the causes of symptoms.

Focal psychodynamic therapy – This is offered when the patient doesn't feel that the above therapies are right for them or if they haven't proved effective. It should include trying to understand how eating habits are related to your thinking, and how the person feels generally about themselves and the people in their life.

MANTRA[18] – This specialist integrative therapy has been developed to address the cognitive, emotional, relational and biological factors related to anorexia. It helps people work out what is keeping them stuck in their anorexia, and then find alternative and more adaptive ways of coping. MANTRA is generally recommended for people who report an extremely rigid thinking style, low motivation for recovery and either no support network or one that they don't feel is helpful.

Diet advice – Advice is given on healthy eating and diet, ideally in combination with talking therapy. Doctors normally also advise people to take vitamin and mineral supplements to ensure they're getting all the nutrients they need to be healthy.

TREATMENT FOR CHILDREN AND YOUNG PEOPLE

Children and young people will usually be offered family therapy, CBT or adolescent-focused psychotherapy. The CBT will be very similar to that offered to adults.

Family therapy involves the person and their family talking to a therapist, exploring how anorexia has affected them and how their family can support them. The therapist will also help them to find ways to manage difficult feelings and situations, aiming to prevent them from relapsing into unhealthy eating habits once the therapy ends.

Adolescent-focused psychotherapy usually lasts between 12 and 18 months. The therapist will help the young person cope with their fears about gaining weight, understand what people need to be healthy and the effects of under-eating, and talk about what's causing the anorexia and how to stop it.

BRIDGING INTERNAL AND EXTERNAL WORLDS

Eating disorders can have a negative impact on people's relationships with family and friends, and on their work and education. They may be linked to depression, low self-esteem, alcohol misuse and self-harm.

The binge/purge cycles associated with bulimia can dominate daily life and lead to difficulties in relationships and social situations. In BED, binges may be planned like a ritual, involving the person buying certain binge foods. People with BED often have feelings of guilt and disgust at their lack of control during and after binge eating, and this may reinforce the cycle of negative emotions, restriction and binge eating.

Social cognitive processes help us to move between our internal thoughts and the outside social world. The way we think about others plays a major role in how we feel about, and interact with, the world around us. Research into social cognition has studied how people process, store and apply information about other people and social situations. This focuses on the role of cognitive processes in our social interactions. These processes are crucial to eating disorders, which bring together social influences around food, weight and diet with our own thinking patterns around these subjects and, more generally, around reward.

Until recently, most of the work in this area relied upon subjective data, where people with eating disorders report on how they think in social situations. Research is now using more objective tests to investigate important aspects of social cognition, such as mentalising, empathy and imitation. Mentalising is the ability to deduce what others are thinking; empathy is the degree to which the emotional states of others can be identified and how much the states of others impact on one's own emotional state; and imitation is the degree to which observation of another's actions prompts the performance of those actions.

Research demonstrates that people with eating disorders are different in how they infer what others think compared to people without eating disorders.[19] They display less imitation of observed actions than those without eating disorders, but there appears to be no difference in empathy. Focusing on processes like this, which span the internal and the external, social world, may reveal opportunities to improve eating disorder treatments.

SUPPORTING TREATMENTS

Treating eating disorders is notoriously challenging and quite often involves the individual moving from inpatient to outpatient services. The transition from being in a very controlled environment, where healthcare workers are providing set meals and weight targets, to trying to maintain positive eating and exercise behaviours at home can be a difficult one. Research involving people with lived experience is enabling a better understanding of the major challenges to treatment and helping to identify approaches to supporting people more effectively.

Once people have had an eating disorder for some time, they usually develop social problems that can make it difficult for them to engage in treatment and develop relationships with staff. Research has demonstrated that healthcare workers' reactions and behaviour towards patients can either impair or facilitate recovery. Similarly, the way in which family members and carers respond to a relation with an eating disorder can play a major role in their recovery and/or the maintenance of their eating disorder.

The concept of 'expressed emotion' is used when discussing schizophrenia, but it also has relevance to eating disorders. Expressed emotion is a measure of the family environment, based on how relatives talk spontaneously about the patient, and includes aspects such as critical comments, hostility, emotional over-involvement, positivity and warmth. These elements are also thought to be relevant for anorexia outcomes. At one end of the spectrum, people may be overprotective, thereby accommodating the illness, while at the other end they may be directly and constantly challenging.

Researchers and clinicians have held workshops for carers in order to help them understand these possible barriers, and share some of the skills that professionals on inpatient units have developed to overcome them. These include how to interview and manage people who are ambivalent about change, and how to enable them to recognise emotions by teaching emotional intelligence.

These workshops have been revisited and improved and the resulting programme is called Experienced Carers Helping Others (ECHO).[20] Researchers are now looking at how similar resources might be developed for BED, which is also a very isolating condition, but in different ways. Different forms of social support may be required that work more on the patient's impulsiveness and what switches them from being in control to out of control.[21]

'I have found the insight of people with lived experience very helpful in our research. This has led to the development of treatments, sharing of skills and materials with patients, and the creation of training and workshops to develop carers' skills. We're trying to create a network where we can all support one other as much as possible and where we're all working on the same page.'

PROFESSOR JANET TREASURE

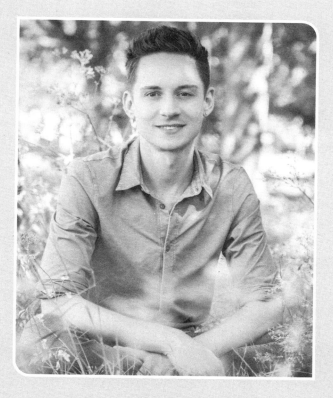

James Downs is a writer, yogi, mental health campaigner and expert by experience in eating disorders. He is an associate lecturer for the Open University, a peer researcher, and a patient representative at the Royal College of Psychiatrists.

It's hard to pinpoint a time when I became ill. I can't identify one event or one specific cause among the whole range of factors. Instead there seem to be several strands that came together

I'm 33 now and I was diagnosed with anorexia when I was 15 but I had signs of disordered eating before then. I'm only now making sense of why and how it happened. In my twenties I developed bulimia and I have now been diagnosed with ADHD, autism, and Ehlers-Danlos syndrome, which is a genetic hypermobility condition. Finding out that I have these conditions has helped me to understand why I've experienced what I've experienced.

CHANGING ENVIRONMENTS

As a young child I felt like I was somehow 'different' from other children, but happy. I wasn't interested in playing with others, but I was happy in my own imaginary world and everyone let me be different. But when I went to high school it was a big change: I started to feel like the ways in which I was different somehow weren't acceptable any more, and I found it difficult to fit in. On a sensory basis it was extremely overwhelming to go from a small, friendly school into a massive comprehensive high school. I found it difficult to navigate this hostile social world.

I think I tried to minimise the sense of feeling threatened and overwhelmed by shutting down my body so I didn't have to feel the pain. When I went to school I wouldn't eat or drink to try to suppress my sensitivity, and when I went home I would eat and drink like normal and my body would come back to life. I realised that I could shut down my body for those experiences that I didn't like, and reawaken it again when it felt safe to do so. For me, the body is the vehicle for all of our experiences – our feelings are felt experiences in the body. When my experience of the world was painful, depriving my body meant I could dial down the pain and not experience it with such intensity.

WEARING AN EATING DISORDER

After a few years, I started to skip school. I was skiving for nearly a year before anybody noticed and when they did I was referred to CAMHS. At that point I had a normal weight, so I wasn't diagnosed with an eating disorder, but I was diagnosed with OCD and depression. Looking back, I think my desire for repetition and familiarity brought about from the undiagnosed ADHD and autism I was living with was mistaken for OCD. Because I was a very bright child with good grades and had learnt how to communicate and pretend to fit in, the professionals seemed to think I would be fine with a few sessions of CBT and go on to live a successful life. But I think this meant that my underlying distress and sense of loneliness and difference were overlooked, and I didn't know how else to communicate them.

This is when the eating disorder kicked in. The professionals seemed so interested in the fact I wasn't eating at school, and would talk about eating disorders as something that they seemed to take very seriously, at the same time as I was feeling like nobody was taking me seriously. The idea of an eating disorder seemed like a solution to me. I couldn't seem to communicate how serious my distress was, but perhaps an eating disorder like anorexia would help me to get the response that I so desperately wanted. This is a controversial point because I don't think it is helpful to think about eating disorders as a choice but, in a way, I think I chose to have anorexia. I remember deciding to lose weight to show how unwell I felt underneath. It wasn't a lifestyle choice or a straightforward choice, and perhaps it wasn't really a choice at all. It was a solution that presented itself to me when I didn't really have any others. Instead of emerging from within me, anorexia was an identity that I could wear, something that I put on, that helped me to make sense of the confusing interactions of help-seeking that I had so far felt like I had failed to navigate. At a time when I had a very uncertain sense of myself and had to leave school – with no friends to work out the messy process of becoming an adult with – anorexia was a very coherent identity that I could inhabit or perform, and, even if it was extremely dangerous, it made sense.

VARIED EXPERIENCES AND ASSUMPTIONS

I think there are lots of assumptions people make about eating disorders – from the kinds of people who experience them to the types of experiences that they have. But there is no one size fits all. I've never had an 'anorexic voice' in my head, and didn't have half of the problems I experienced with anorexia at the start until I learnt that the identity of 'being anorexic' meant I had to become preoccupied with my body shape, over-exercise and use more and more extreme means to lose weight. It also frustrates me when people say that eating disorders are all about 'control', because in my experience it's often been about control in order to feel safe, not control in and of itself. When we feel safe, we don't feel the need to be in control, and we can let go. I struggled to find that opportunity, and many of the people who were supposed to help me with the eating disorder didn't help me to first feel safe enough to try to change.

People also thought that I would grow out of anorexia when I came to terms with being gay, but to me this felt like another lazy assumption and perhaps even a way to not have to provide care for me. I was also told from a young age that I would never recover and that eating disorders are conditions people will always have in some way. Being told this before I had even had treatment filled me with despair and the evidence just isn't there to show that people don't recover from eating disorders – they don't recover because of a lack of treatment.

Being a male with an eating disorder I've also felt quite fetishised, like a rare specimen for professionals to gawp at. When it comes to increasing the diversity of experiences we consider when we think about eating disorders, making special categories isn't the answer and can feel even more stigmatising. Instead, we need to hear a whole range of stories from people of different backgrounds as though they are normal and expected, not shocking or somehow alien.

TAKING A NEW APPROACH

At the moment, I am undertaking cognitive analytic therapy and, although it hasn't helped me to change my behaviours yet, it has been useful in understanding how I have different states of health and how my physical and mental health conditions interact as a whole. I inhabit very different states in my life – from being very high-functioning and performative where I do a lot of public speaking, teaching, yoga, dance and music, to being in a state of feeling unwell, which is completely invisible to the outside world. In this state I'm often struggling with my health and unable to communicate it to others, which can make me distressed and increasingly unwell and isolated. It feels like a trap that I am unable to get out of because bulimia will kick in to cope with the difficult feelings and disarm me from my ability to speak out and reach out to others. Sometimes it feels as if I don't want to exist for a while and I want to destroy that time and then the bulimia steps in and fills that time and I almost dissociate from the world. Like most things, the solution is about finding balance, and at the moment I am working out how to inhabit a new space or identity, between these two states.

I didn't have specialist treatment or therapy for eating disorders until six and a half years after my diagnosis. I wish I had been assessed for neurodevelopmental conditions and Ehlers-Danlos syndrome earlier, and am still shocked at how many things were overlooked simply because I was a compliant and intelligent child who was able to learn how to get by and not complain. I often think about how things could have been different, but recovery for me can't ever be about going back to a time before I was unwell, or reclaiming things I have lost. Instead, I have to try to discover something new.

CO-CREATING KNOWLEDGE OF EATING DISORDERS TOGETHER

I am encouraged by the growing inclusion of the voices of people with lived experience of eating disorders in research and the development of treatments. I have been very involved in co-production work and this is at its best when I am not just asked for advice but have been a key part of the decision-making process. Not only has it been personally affirming and increased my confidence and skills to take part in research, it also helps to redress imbalances in terms of who gets to decide what we know about eating disorders. This feels like a bit of justice for all of those times when I have not felt listened to or like I have had a say in my own treatment.

I think eating disorders – and all mental health problems – are biological, social and psychological. We think of them as very discrete categories, and I have spent many years being told that everything is 'all in my head' when in fact I have had underlying physiological problems. The experiences of people like me who have eating disorders and another condition such as hypermobility or autism show that the systems of the body, mind and society are all interconnected.

I think of it like a mosaic: all these pieces that shift and then the environment will change but there might be some underlying constancy in our biology or sensitivities. I think diagnostic categories are quite blinding and eating disorders are narrowly defined, both in terms of the condition and also in terms of treatment and recovery. We need to be more creative – from creating new knowledge about eating disorders to creating new ways of responding to them to help people create the lives they deserve to have.

THE ROLE OF APPETITE AND PARENTING

Appetite, and the mechanisms that influence how we react to food and how much food we can eat, have been examined in connection with obesity. Different aspects of appetite can be studied from a very early age, providing an insight into who might be most likely to become obese and enabling treatments to be put in place earlier on. There has, however, been little investigation into the importance of appetite in eating disorders. Researchers are now trying to examine appetite as an avenue to both identifying those at risk of developing an eating disorder and understanding the mechanisms behind these conditions.

The word 'appetite' tends to be used positively in our culture, so we'll talk about children having a 'good' or 'healthy' appetite. In research, however, the concept of appetite is multifaceted, with various mechanisms and ways to measure them. It is not 'good' or 'bad', but rather a continuum of variations that can be monitored and related to our physical and mental health. Two broad concepts used in appetite research are food and satiety responsiveness.

Food responsiveness is the urge to eat when you see, smell or taste food that is palatable and attractive. Research has shown that children who react more strongly to appetising food than others are more likely to become overweight later on in life.[22]

The concept of satiety is often described as 'being full' and satiety responsiveness is a person's sensitivity to being full. We study this as a means to understanding how we regulate intake of food in relation to being full. Research has shown that children who take longer to feel full, or who have a tendency to ignore this feeling, tend to get heavier over time.[23]

'How we, as parents and carers, respond to our children's behaviour and emotions, and whether we use food as part of this response, can turn food into something far more complex than fuel and nutrition. We may, unintentionally, attach new meanings to food in terms of emotions and rewards, and this may, in turn, impact how children's eating behaviours develop. On top of that, we live in an environment where we are surrounded by food and food cues. There are constant conversations about dieting habits, new diets and so-called "fat talk", when adults complain about their weight or talk about other people gaining weight in a negative way. All this influences how we feel about, and behave around, food.'

PROFESSOR CLARE LLEWELLYN

Researchers propose that genes influence our weight through these appetite-related mechanisms. This is because our genetic make-up governs our gut hormones, and how our physiology responds to food and opportunities to eat in the context of a very strong gene environment interaction. Someone who inherits a set of genes that makes them very responsive to food cues and who is not protected by strong satiety (i.e. they have weak sensitivity to fullness) will be very food responsive. In the current environment, such individuals are particularly susceptible to obesity. In comparison, an individual who has inherited a set of genes that gives them low interest in food and high sensitivity to satiety will be protected from obesity, whatever environment they live in. This is called behavioural susceptibility.[24]

PARENTING, ENVIRONMENT AND GENES

Parental factors can also play an important role in the development of eating behaviours. This influence is bidirectional, so the parents react to their child's behaviour around food and the child responds to their parents' behaviour in return. In the same way that they might give a child who loves reading more books, a parent will tend to offer food to a child if it seems to soothe them or they enjoy it. Children who are more responsive to food send more of these signals to their parents. Often, food also has an emotional connection, so parents will use a favourite food as a reward or distraction, or withhold it as a punishment. Although parenting is considered an environmental influence, rather than genetic, parental practices around food can be passed down through the generations and remain within families for years.

Research has shown that parental response can lead to an increase in food responsiveness and that, over time, this can nurture emotional overeating. Studies are now exploring whether early patterns in appetite, and other factors relating to the home feeding environment, might act as indicators of eating disorders. One of the challenges of such research is that there are relatively few people who go on to develop eating disorders, so drawing firm conclusions about any relationships is difficult. This can be overcome by amalgamating a number of datasets that follow people over time.

Having looked at the link between different aspects of appetite and weight and or obesity, researchers are now asking the question as to whether the same mechanisms are involved in eating disorders and if it is possible to identify risk factors from early patterns in appetite and parental factors. Studies using data from multiple longitudinal twin studies, including Gemini, TEDS and Generation R,[25] have tracked mental health, genetic and parental factors from birth through to teenage years. The findings could be used to inform parents on healthy eating practices and offer early detection of eating disorders through screening programmes. Ultimately, this work will provide new knowledge about the emergence of these conditions, and how we might prevent them from developing.

The role of genetics in appetite is another area of interest, especially as it is thought to be closely linked to our evolutionary response to food availability. One approach that is often used to try to disentangle the influences of our genes and environment is the study of twins, and the comparison of identical and non-identical twins. Another approach attempts to distinguish which environmental aspects among twins are completely shared, such as parental feeding and food availability in the home, and which are unique to the individual, such as friends and past bouts of illness. By looking at these different aspects of the environment and comparing them between twins it is possible to make some conclusions about the influence of shared or individual factors on eating.

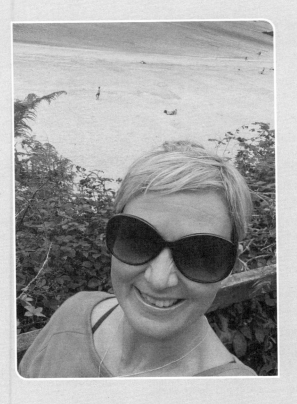

Jo Fort is a senior manager in the NHS secondary care system, working at some of the busiest NHS trusts in central England. She has spent many hours juggling budgets, and dealing with one crisis after another, finding effective solutions to problems so patients have easy access to the best healthcare. But being a mum and understanding and *navigating a pathway for her own daughter was even more important. She didn't have the ability to fix but managed to find ways to help.*

Annie wasn't formally diagnosed until May this year when she was 20 but it started before then. The build-up was maybe a year before in terms of the gradual loss of confidence and becoming very self-conscious about her appearance. Then she self-harmed badly on her arm and leg and it turns out she'd done it before.

Around that time she asked to use my fitness pal, which counts your calorie intake and expenditure. I thought she was just interested in being healthy but then she told me that she was feeling guilty if she ate cakes. I didn't think it was serious because a lot of women and girls struggle with weight and feeling guilty after they eat. But then – I remember it distinctly – when we were at a social event a family member commented that they thought she'd put some weight on her face . . .

I remember seeing the look on her face and I knew at that point that I'd lost her. I just knew it. She asked her friend to pick her up and she messaged me to say it had really affected her and she wasn't sure she could get past it. So we started researching and we went on the Beat website and got some online counselling support and although she hadn't lost a lot of weight at this point, they said that it wasn't the case that you have to lose weight for it to be an eating disorder. They said she had a disordered relationship with food and that's enough.

SEEKING HELP

It was when we were going away for a weekend and Annie told me that she didn't think she was well and needed help. She knew I was trying to support but she said it felt like we were brushing the problem under the carpet. So we got an appointment with the GP but it was over the phone and he said he didn't think she had an eating disorder because she hadn't lost weight. And, thinking back, this is one of the worst things you can say to someone who is in the early stages, but he did refer her because of the previous self-harm.

So we managed to get a referral to the FREED team, which is an early intervention eating disorder team for adults. They said the next available appointment was in about two months – and I knew this meant Annie wouldn't think she was sick enough and that she was going to make sure that between that time and the appointment she would make it clear that she was ill – and that's exactly what happened.

ANOREXIC VOICE

Eating disorders are so complex and many people have what is called an anorexic voice. This voice is in their head all the time telling them that they're greedy, they're fat, they're ugly, they're not deserving, they're not sick enough, they're not thin enough . . . And ultimately what the illness wants to do is kill them. Annie was at the start of that journey but she'd already got that voice. It was where the guilt was coming from and it just took a bigger hold and the voice in her head told her that if she didn't lose weight they weren't going to take her seriously. So, between the beginning of January and her assessment in March she went from 48 kilos to 43 kilos, which is the borderline between being a healthy weight and starting to be underweight.

She started to put in place all these rules around eating. Anorexia is very rule-driven and people set themselves parameters that don't have any rationale but that make sense to them and make them feel safe. People with anorexia talk a lot about having safe foods, and over the course of those two months Annie cut a lot of different foods out of her diet. Breakfast and lunch became fixed.

Breakfast was always cornflakes with no sugar and a tiny bit of milk. For lunch she would only eat these protein bagels so I was always panicking when I went to the supermarket in case they didn't have them in stock, because if they didn't have them she wouldn't eat anything.

BEING A PARENT

I started reading a lot about the subject and everything described the role of being a parent as being to re-feed your child. It's the parents' responsibility to increase calorie intake because professionals aren't at home and they're not the person cooking for them. But the problem is how do you get somebody to eat who doesn't want to eat . . . and when 'not eating' is the driving force of the illness.

It's really difficult. I still don't know how to do it, and I don't know how parents whose children are hospitalised manage to do it. If they don't want to eat they won't eat. For a long time I had to get Annie her breakfast and her lunch or she wouldn't eat anything. And I had to prove to her that the grams in her cereal were what they should be otherwise she wouldn't accept it.

I would stay with her when she ate. There's a lot of evidence showing that sitting close to somebody who's got anorexia and making them feel safe or using distraction techniques can help. So we used to sit and do a word game on her phone. Annie became obsessed with cookery programmes and her mind became completely and utterly absorbed by food. It's not that she didn't want to eat, but she couldn't allow herself to eat. So she obsessed about everything that she wasn't letting herself do.

And you really can't cheat when you give them food. Annie was so aware and if she asked me what's in this or how many calories does this food contain I couldn't lie to her because I was so scared that if she found out I would lose her trust. So I've never lied to her because trust is everything. And we were really fortunate because anorexia is an incredibly deceitful, horrible, isolating illness that makes people feel shameful and guilty. A lot of anorexic sufferers don't talk to people because they feel so ashamed. So I feel quite privileged that Annie actually trusted me enough to talk to me about it, because that's quite unusual. It doesn't mean that she hasn't had those feelings but it does mean that she recognised that she needed help and needed to talk.

IMPACT ON FAMILY

At the start I was a bit of an emotional wreck and I went on antidepressants to try to level that out. After Annie's assessment with FREED I gave up work because she was saying it would be better for her and for everybody else if she wasn't here any more. I couldn't go to work and function knowing this was how she felt.

My husband was really worried about me and how it was impacting us as a family. Annie's brother really struggled and then you have to deal with everybody's else's views on eating disorders and try to educate people who don't understand. In particular my mum and dad have always seen a lot of Annie but she withdrew from them and, when she did see them, my mum got really emotional and often said the wrong thing, which can have a dramatic impact. So I spent time trying to educate my mum and dad and explaining that Annie might want to bring her own food if we go somewhere and try not to draw attention if she did.

RECOVERY JOURNEY

When we got a new GP it was the first time anybody had actually physically sat in front of Annie and given her validation. Just hearing that somebody believes her and wants to help her is hugely significant and, for me as parent, knowing that somebody is looking after her physical health is really important because I was terrified. It's all I could think about. I was terrified that my child was going to die and that every day they get worse it's another day that's harder to get them better. So you are so desperate for intervention and for somebody to take control and as a parent your instinct is to just protect your child at any cost.

The hardest thing was coming to terms with the fact that I couldn't make her better. I didn't have the ability to fix this but I managed to find ways to help, I learnt how to listen properly. I think most of us think we're good listeners but when you are *really* listening, you are reflecting back what they're saying and not trying to take control. And this is really difficult because Annie regressed quite a lot, which is quite common.

I came to realise that, although she couldn't do it on her own, ultimately the change had to come from her, and it did. There came a time when she wanted to get better and realised she had to do it and that was the pivotal change.

She's come such a long way and I've come to accept that this is a massive journey. It's not something that gets fixed overnight or in a couple of months. I think once you come to terms with this then you can learn to live with it in a different way. What's important is that it doesn't totally consume you and for Annie a huge part of her recovery is understanding that she doesn't need to have anorexia to be validated even if that's what her anorexia tells her.

There's no actual cure to anorexia. Some people do fully recover and go on to lead normal lives and some recover by learning how to manage it. But I think it's very difficult to really truly lift this obsession with food. Society and social media have a huge responsibility for this and I've become much more aware of trying to be accepting of who you are as a person and what you look like. That's what I want to teach Annie because I look at her and just see this beautiful person who's nearly been destroyed by a horrible illness but is fighting her way through.

TWIN STUDY ON APPETITE

Research has examined how food and satiety responsiveness are distinct in their influence on eating patterns.[26] The study involved 2,203 toddlers from Gemini, a large study of families with twins born in the UK in 2007. When the children were 16 months old, parents completed a questionnaire about their food and satiety responsiveness and kept food and drink diaries over three days.

The study found that food and satiety responsiveness led to different eating patterns. Children who were very responsive to food cues ate more often, and those less sensitive to fullness consumed more calories each time they ate. These findings suggest that, while both food responsiveness and satiety responsiveness may lead to overeating, they do so in different ways.

Food, for many people, is in abundant supply, easily accessible and widely advertised. As a result, children who are highly responsive to food have many opportunities to act on their urges to eat. A child who takes longer to feel full, or is less sensitive to signs of being full, is also likely to eat more at a meal in order to feel satisfied. The study shows that some children are better at regulating their appetites than others, with those who have a weaker food response and stronger satiety response doing it in different ways.

CURRENT AND FUTURE DEVELOPMENTS

EARLY INTERVENTION

Often, eating disorders develop early in life and become more entrenched and difficult to challenge as people grow older. Many report that their condition started as a way of dealing with difficult emotions. There is, therefore, a window of opportunity early on in people's lives, where eating disorders may be prevented from becoming ingrained and where the emotional difficulties that accompany them may be addressed.

Approaches such as First Episode Rapid Early Intervention for Eating Disorders (FREED)[27] have been developed to this effect. FREED is a service available to 16–25-year-olds, giving them rapid access to specialised treatment in the first three years of their eating disorder. Evidence shows that changes to the brain, body and behaviour are more easily reversed in these first three years.

One challenge is that, in order for early intervention to work in practice, people need to be aware of their condition and willing to receive treatment. This is particularly difficult for young people when they leave home and are no longer surrounded by their families. Student Minds, a UK mental health charity, is working to increase awareness around eating disorders and provide advice on peer support. Such work needs to happen in tandem with a shift in society's awareness and perception of eating disorders.

'We have to remember that any guidelines or advice around eating practices have to be very sensitively worded. Parents should never be made to feel guilty if their child develops eating difficulties.'

PROFESSOR CLARE LLEWELLYN

'I would like to see the development of an early-life intervention that is successful in reducing the number of adolescents who develop eating disorders symptoms. However, there would have to be complex interventions. There also needs to be a wider collective responsibility at a community level as we need to change the way we talk about body size, weight and calories. It needs to be something incorporated into the school curriculum.'

PROFESSOR CLARE LEWELLYN

MULTIDISCIPLINARY APPROACH

Eating disorders are complex, with many factors influencing how they begin, develop and are maintained. They are also long-lasting conditions, with far-reaching impacts on the people experiencing them, as well as on their families and friends. While they are challenging to treat, with better understanding and a multidisciplinary approach, it is certainly possible.

Experts in genetics, brain imaging, cognitive science and social psychology are just some of those who could contribute to the research and development of treatments. Most importantly, perhaps, experts with lived experience can provide their vital insight into living with eating disorders. Work also needs to take place in the realm of public health to remove the stigma surrounding eating disorders, raise awareness and address our often unhealthy societal conversations around food. This work could help to unlock the potential for research and enable treatments to have a greater impact.

Research has shown a linear association between childhood obesity and neighbourhood deprivation. This suggests that when people are born with a predisposition to react to food in a certain way, it can translate into obesity if they live in a household with no access to healthy food and are bombarded with food cues. Despite this, the general public belief is still that it's entirely within someone's remit to control their weight.

NOVEL TREATMENTS

New treatments in development are trying to shift the ingrained patterns of thinking that appear to be instrumental in the maintenance of these long-lasting conditions. These treatments include hormones, psychedelics, AVATAR therapy and non-invasive brain stimulation.

TREATING HORMONE IMBALANCE

The behavioural symptoms of anorexia are linked to those of starvation, which develop after a prolonged restriction of food intake. Research has shown that when levels of fat fall, there is also a drop in levels of the adipocyte hormone leptin in the blood. This signals to the body to adapt to starvation, causing symptoms such as cessation of periods, changes in the blood composition, depressed mood and constant thoughts of food. Another behaviour often linked to low levels of leptin is hyperactivity. It has been suggested that this, and possibly other symptoms related to starvation in anorexia, may be alleviated by treatment with metreleptin, which is a manufactured chemical version of leptin. Research on small numbers of patients with anorexia found that treatment with metreleptin can reduce the desire for activity, repetitive thoughts of food, inner restlessness and weight phobia.[28] It is likely that this approach would work best with those patients shown to have low levels of leptin in the blood.

VIRTUAL REALITY AND AVATAR THERAPY

The AVATAR therapy approach was first developed to treat psychosis. People are able to create a computerised representation of the voices they hear as a way to challenge and have some control over them. Research is looking at the feasibility of implementing an adapted form of AVATAR therapy to reduce the power of the eating disorder voice.[29] Having created the avatar of their eating disorder voice, the patient can provide examples of the kinds of comments it might make. In the company of a therapist, they can then interact with the avatar, standing up to the critical comments it makes in order to develop a sense of power, control and self-awareness.

PSYCHEDELICS

Psilocybin is a controlled drug and a constituent of so-called 'magic mushrooms'. It produces a range of subjective effects, including altering the way that things look and sometimes eliciting emotional insights and visions. Recent studies suggest that psilocybin may have a role in managing conditions such as depression, addiction and obsessive compulsive disorder through its action on the serotonin system in the brain. In particular, it has been trialled on people who are resistant to other treatments. It is thought that psilocybin enables people to shift from their entrenched thinking patterns, and research is looking to test whether it might be helpful in treating anorexia nervosa. Participants in this research will be supported by a therapist throughout the experience and it is hoped psilocybin will have the potential to shift thinking patterns and behaviour in those who have had anorexia for a long time.

NON-INVASIVE BRAIN STIMULATION (NIBS)

A better understanding of the brain processes involved in eating disorders has enabled more targeted, brain-directed treatments to be developed. Non-invasive brain stimulation (NIBS), such as repetitive transcranial magnetic stimulation (rTMS) and transcranial direct current stimulation (tDCS), allows safe, pain-free stimulation of specific brain areas using magnetic fields and electrical currents, respectively.

NIBS is being used increasingly to treat a range of psychiatric disorders, and early studies in eating disorders have shown that it can improve eating behaviours and mood. Research has primarily targeted the dorsolateral prefrontal cortex (DLPFC), an area of the brain involved in controlling social/emotional reactions and cognitive processes, such as planning and decision-making, and in inhibiting unhelpful behaviours.

A clinical trial of rTMS[30] to the prefrontal cortex has already taken place on patients with severe enduring anorexia nervosa. The procedure resulted in major early improvements in mood and quality of life. In the longer term, 45.5 per cent of patients who received rTMS reached a BMI at which they were no longer considered anorexic, compared to only 9 per cent of those in the group who did not receive the treatment. Using brain imaging, researchers found after rTMS a significant decrease in activity in the amygdala, a part of the brain involved in fear and stress.[31] This was related to reduced patient-reported anxiety/stress and unhelpful behaviours towards food.[32] Researchers are now trialling a variant of rTMS in young people with treatment-resistant anorexia nervosa and are exploring the use of non-invasive brain stimulation in the treatment of bulimic disorders. This is being combined with cognitive training to maximise effects.

SPOTLIGHT ON GENETIC COUNSELLING IN MENTAL HEALTH

There is increasing interest in the role of genes and the environment in mental health conditions. When we talk about 'environment' it can encompass a range of different factors, from early childhood experiences and how we were raised to our social relationships, and our surrounding culture. Research with twins has shown that our genetic make-up is more influential for some mental health conditions than others: for example, schizophrenia and autism spectrum disorder have a stronger genetic basis than conditions such as depression and anxiety. What is now generally recognised is that for all conditions it is not a question of genes OR environment but a discussion around the complex interplay between the two.

'It's about trying to resolve some of the emotional baggage that we carry around with our mental illness in terms of guilt, shame, blame, fear, stigma – all these things that people attach to their explanations for the cause of illness. I believe that's how you can make progress in terms of engaging people in behaviour changes that might help protect their mental health for the future. If I was to distil it down all into one sentence, really what we're doing in genetic counselling for psychiatric illness is helping people to understand this is not their fault but there might be ways we can better protect their mental health for the future.'

PROFESSOR JEHANNINE AUSTIN

Researchers are now applying novel techniques and harnessing large datasets to tease apart the complex interactions between our genes and our environment. At a finer level we are discovering more from the field of epigenetics about the mechanisms that govern this interaction. Not only is this providing a more in-depth picture of mental health that can inform treatments, but this knowledge can directly provide a platform to help people reach their own understanding about what underlies their mental health and, based on this, think about their life decisions.

Genetic counselling is a relatively new approach to healthcare and involves helping individuals and families who have, or who are at risk of, conditions that have a genetic component to understand and adapt to the medical, psychological and familial implications of the disease or condition. The process involves:

Interpretation of family and medical histories to assess the chance of disease occurrence or recurrence

Education about inheritance, testing, management, prevention and resources

Counselling to promote informed choices and adaptation to the risk or condition

The approach has been used for some time for rare hereditary physical conditions such as cystic fibrosis, Duchenne muscular dystrophy and haemophilia, but its application to psychiatric disorders is relatively new. By considering the genetic contribution to a mental health condition, the counselling approach enables individuals to think about how these conditions can result from the combination of experiences and genes and, through this, how best they can manage their mental health for the future.

TOOLS OF GENETIC COUNSELLING

Mental Illness Jar

One of the tools that has been developed by genetic counsellors in psychiatric conditions is the 'mental illness jar', to represent a person's mental health state. The concept proposes that when people experience an episode of illness, the jar is filled to the top. Different people's jars can become filled with different quantities of genetic and environmental (or experiential) vulnerability factors. An environmental factor might be job stress, financial concerns, family issues or personal loss.

Importantly, what the concept of the mental illness jar shows (and which accurately reflects research findings) is that we ALL

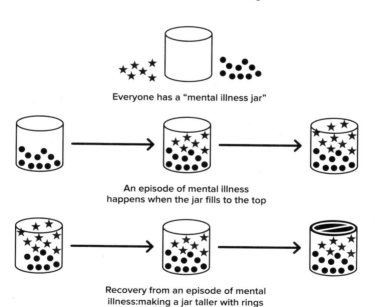

Everyone has a "mental illness jar"

An episode of mental illness
happens when the jar fills to the top

Recovery from an episode of mental
illness:making a jar taller with rings

●   Genetic vulnerability factor
★   Environmental vulnerability factor
◉   Protective factor

MENTAL ILLNESS JAR

have some genetic vulnerability to mental illness, and that genetic vulnerability doesn't change. However, we can make ourselves more resilient to mental illness through identifying and putting in place protective factors; this is represented by making the jar taller by 'stacking rings' on top of it. This creates more room for environmental factors and slows down the speed at which the jar fills up. Some of these rings or protective factors (like sleep, nutrition, exercise and good social support) are good for all of us, regardless of our genes. However, some protective factors can be more individual. In Alastair's story in Chapter 1 he talks about his use of the mental illness jar and cites football, learning a language and the city of Burnley as the rings or protective factors.

By using this mental illness jar and other tools, genetic counsellors can play an important role in helping people process the emotions they're facing that can be associated with health conditions they're living with. Using the findings of scientific research about the interplay between genetics and environment, they shape an approach that can help people explore their understanding of their condition. Below are two examples of concepts based in scientific research that can be used by genetic counsellors: epigenetics and polygenic scores.

EPIGENETICS

Epigenetics is a field of science that explores how your experiences can cause changes that affect the way your genes work. Unlike genetic changes, epigenetic changes are reversible and do not change your DNA sequence, but they can change how your body reads a DNA sequence. This can be a useful concept to use in genetic counselling, and the complex mechanism behind epigenetics can be represented relatively simply in the mental illness jar.

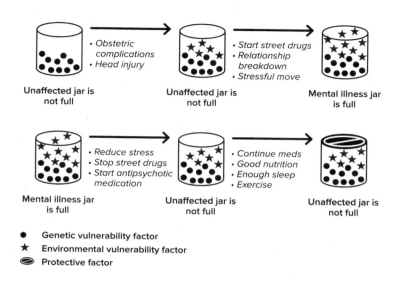

- Genetic vulnerability factor
★ Environmental vulnerability factor
◉ Protective factor

THE MENTAL ILLNESS JAR

For example, people can have an unusual genetic factor in their jar that has a relatively small influence in isolation but can, in the presence of a particular environmental aspect or influence, suddenly produce a large impact on mental health. In the picture of the mental health jar this is when the star fills up the space instead of just remaining small, meaning the effect of the environment is disproportionately large for people who have a particular genetic variation. This can also work in the other direction; so the impact of environmental influence might usually be small, but if there is a specific genetic make-up then it will have a much bigger effect.

POLYGENIC SCORES

Genetic influence in psychiatric conditions is not simple. There are a range of different kinds of genetic contributions that can play a role in a person's vulnerability to developing psychiatric

'How I see polygenic scores is as a way to open up a conversation around what they think about their mental health so that I can help people feel less anxious, afraid, guilty or ashamed about their mental health issues so this no longer prevents them from trying to implement changes in their life that might help them in the long run. It's about using what we know about genetics and the environment to find a way to empower people.'

PROFESSOR JEHANNINE AUSTIN

illness. Some of these contributions are very small: for example, the smallest possible units of DNA, which are called single nucleotide polymorphisms (SNPs). Individually these tiny, single blocks have infinitesimally small effects but, as there are hundreds of different SNPs, if you put them all together then that is the level of where impact can happen. Such diseases and disorders have what is called a 'polygenic' underpinning, where instead of only one gene or a few playing a role in the risk of diseases, it is likely that thousands of genes are having an effect; inherited changes in each gene make a modest impact on our risk of each disease.

A polygenic score brings together the many, tiny different genetic changes in a person that can influence their vulnerability to psychiatric illness. Most people will have a score that is near average, but a few people will have a high polygenic score, putting them at increased risk of developing a particular disease.

Polygenic scores are potentially valuable ways to understand our mental health and potentially guide our behaviours to develop more protective factors but currently they are not being used directly in clinical practice. Part of the reason is even the best polygenic score that we can generate explains only a very small fraction of a person's overall chance of developing psychiatric illness – so even with a high polygenic score, a person may still not develop the condition.

GENETIC COUNSELLING IN PREGNANCY

The time before and after having a child (the perinatal period) is a risk period for mental illness. It is a period of profound change, whether that be change that is exciting and positive or change that is stressful. For those who have a history of mental illness there is a greater chance of developing psychiatric problems in this period,[33] but there is limited data on the risks associated with taking psychotropic medications during pregnancy[34] as it is very difficult to conduct clinical trials on pregnant women. However, there is also risk – for both mother and baby – associated with untreated mental illness during pregnancy.

The guidelines that exist for clinicians in this area suggest that they should help people make value-based decisions about medication during this time. This is challenging when the data is minimal and many healthcare professionals do not have the time or resources to enable people to work out their values and unpick what feels right for them. Using qualitative interviews, researchers have investigated how women make decisions about antidepressants during pregnancy; the results show that there's a gap in terms of what women need to know so they can feel positive about making these decisions.[35] Genetic counselling is a possible approach to help bridge this gap and provide people with the support they need. For example, research has shown genetic counselling to be a positive experience for women who are due to have an amniocentesis procedure (which assesses whether their foetus has an abnormal number of chromosomes).[36]

The issue of decision-making goes further back, to the initial choice to become pregnant. Women with psychiatric disorders with a known strong genetic component, such as schizophrenia or bipolar disorder, often report having been advised by healthcare providers not to have children because of the possibility of a relapse during or after pregnancy and because of the perceived likelihood that the condition will be inherited by their children. Genetic counsellors however do not endorse this perspective – they do not advise people whether or not to have children; rather, they specialise in promoting and supporting individuals' rights to make autonomous decisions about their own health.

'My perspective on things is that everybody is going to have challenges with parenting. Every single person. Parenting is not easy, it's incredibly hard and if you have a mental illness then you just happen to know what one of your challenges might be before you go into it.'

PROFESSOR JEHANNINE AUSTIN

When people are in a difficult stage of mental illness, they may lose the ability to make a decision for themselves about the future. This is known as losing mental capacity. Research is underway on advance statements, which will enable women to put in place decisions about their future should they have a relapse or need support during pregnancy or when they have their child.

An advance statement or advance decision covering future care and treatment would explain to professionals and loved ones what that person would like to happen in the future. Having this in place can enable people to feel in control of what happens to them. Healthcare professionals can help women write their advance statement when they are pregnant so they can describe what they would like to happen to them and/or their baby if their condition becomes difficult to manage.

'When you're in a good place and you've got insight, it can be so empowering to have a conversation about what you would want to happen if you become unwell. What would you want to happen if you've just delivered a baby and you have a psychotic episode? Having this conversation in advance can give you pre-emptive control for if and when you're sick.'

PROFESSOR JEHANNINE AUSTIN

GENETIC COUNSELLING IN SUBSTANCE USE

Research has shown that substance use and addiction are often closely related to trauma as an experience. Living with trauma can be very painful and in the short term substance use numbs the pain. It may feel like some form of protective factor because it helps people forget the pain of the trauma, but substance use has other consequences that can end up compounding the problems rather than resolving them (see Chapter 3 on PTSD).

Genetic counselling can be helpful for people in terms of building their own self-compassion and considering replacements or alternatives to try to address their mental health needs or their pain.

Taking the specific example of cannabis, research shows a well-established association between cannabis use and psychotic illness such as schizophrenia, but there has been ongoing debate as to which one caused the other – was it the cannabis that made people more vulnerable to developing psychosis or did people with schizophrenia start using cannabis as a way to manage their condition?

Eventually there was a series of studies that demonstrated that it wasn't simply one explanation or another but that both were true. And this is also the case in many other conditions. Large-scale studies with genetic data from saliva swaps such as the UK Biobank, and other projects such as GLAD (Genetic Links to Anxiety and Depression study), are improving our understanding of genetic involvement in mental health. Alongside this, technological developments are allowing individuals to get their own genetic screening. However, our genetic knowledge will always be part of the puzzle of understanding our mental health and not the whole answer.

'It's just a very human response to feeling so hurt – you want the pain to stop, and you try to find what you can to help with that. And it isn't easy to stop using substances because it is all that some people have to manage their hurt – and you need to be able to replace that protection offered by substances with something else.'

PROFESSOR JEHANNINE AUSTIN

WHERE NOW?

One of the key things to remember about eating disorders is that they can affect anyone of any weight. It is a myth that people with eating disorders are always very thin. In fact, anyone with an unhealthy relationship to food could be considered to have an eating disorder.

Binge-eating disorder, bulimia, anorexia and OSFED or 'Other Specified Feeding or Eating Disorder' can affect men and women of any age. Eating disorders can be very dangerous if left untreated; they can cause long-term damage to organs such as the liver and kidneys and can even in extreme cases cause death.

If you are worried about your relationship with food, in the first instance you should speak to your GP. The earlier you seek professional assistance the more likely it is to be effective and to avert long-term bodily harm.

If you are concerned about a loved one, particularly a child or young person, you should encourage them to see their GP. You might even want to accompany them to an appointment.

Your GP will ask about eating habits and feelings and might also do a physical examination including weighing and measuring. Alternatively they may refer you to a specialist who will do this instead.

There are many different types of eating disorders and so there are many different types of treatment. However, one thing is true across the board: the approach taken with young people is usually different to that taken with adults.

Children and adolescents are usually offered family therapy or adolescent-focused CBT.

Family therapy involves the family talking to a therapist. This could be just the child and parents or could include siblings and extended family members such as grandparents. The aim of family therapy is to explore solutions for managing difficult feelings and unhealthy eating habits and to learn how the family can be supportive. Family therapy is usually offered for between 18 and 20 sessions over a year. Waiting lists can be long, so if you are able you may want to explore options for doing this privately.

Adolescent-focused cognitive behavioural therapy (CBT) is a talking therapy usually offered on a one-to-one basis, although sometimes parents are included, and takes place with a specially trained therapist.

For adults, talking and psychological therapies also usually take place on a one-to-one basis. Because there are many different types of talking therapy, it is important that you don't give up if you don't start to feel better straight away. People respond differently to different types of treatment, and even to different therapists. So it is very important that you let your doctor know if you are not feeling any better after around 8–10 weeks of therapy, so that adjustments in treatment can be made.

In some cases, particularly where there are concerns about physical health, diet supplements such as vitamins may be prescribed by your doctor, or they may even recommend that you visit hospital if they feel you need more intensive treatment.

It can be very difficult to recognise that you have an eating disorder, and often it is noticed by loved ones before an individual recognises it themselves. If you are worried about yourself or a loved one, but are not yet ready to speak to your GP, here are some sources of advice and support:

BeatEatingDisorders.org.uk

BEAT offer advice both to people experiencing symptoms of eating disorders and to carers. Their helpline is open 365 days a year from 9am–midnight on weekdays and 4pm–midnight on weekends and bank holidays:

England: 0808 801 0677

Scotland: 0808 801 0432

Wales: 0808 801 0433

Northern Ireland: 0808 801 0434

Nationaleatingdisorders.org

NEDA offer a number of online resources, including a self-screening tool to determine if it's time you reached out for help for disrupted eating.

To find out more about the latest research into eating disorders from MQ, just scan here:

the experts

JANET TREASURE

Janet Treasure is a psychiatrist working at King's College London and South London and Maudsley NHS Foundation Trust who specialises in the research and treatment of eating disorders. She first became aware of eating disorders at the age of 16 when a girl at her school developed anorexia. At the time, little was known about the condition. While she was at medical school one of her peers developed the disease and Janet became more and more interested in the factors underlying its development. She decided to specialise in psychiatry, starting as a locum at the Maudsley Hospital under Gerald Russell – a pioneer in the study of eating disorders – who inspired her interest in research. She received a fellowship to study endocrine factors in anorexia and has combined a research and clinical career ever since. Janet is particularly interested in co-developing, delivering and co-authoring information and interventions together with people with eating disorders and their families. During her career she has seen how views on eating disorders have changed, with treatment and research shifting from the realm of medicine to that of psychiatry, so that now we are at a place where recent genetic findings have brought recognition that risk factors in both the brain and body could be possible targets for treatment. In 2013 she was awarded an OBE for her work in eating disorders and in 2022 she was made a fellow of the Academy of Medical Sciences.

CLARE LLEWELLYN

Clare Llewellyn is an MQ/Rosetrees fellow and Associate Professor of Obesity in the Department of Behavioural Science and Health at University College London, where she leads the Obesity Research Group. Her research interests focus on understanding how genetic and environmental factors interact to influence weight and eating behaviour, and she is now investigating the shared mechanisms between obesity and eating disorders as they first start to emerge in childhood and adolescence. As a child she was a very fussy eater and remembers the stress it caused her and her family. She wishes there had been more awareness around childhood feeding problems at the time, so she and her family could have received more support. Throughout her teens she continued to eat a very limited range of foods, until she shared a house at university, at which point she turned a corner and quickly became much more adventurous with trying new foods. During her psychology undergraduate degree she found herself naturally drawn towards twin studies as a way to understand why people can respond differently to the same event. Initially she was planning on becoming a clinical psychologist but, after taking a module in health psychology, she became very interested in the interface between mental and physical health and this led her to specialise in researching obesity, eating behaviour and eating disorders. She now leads the Gemini Study, the largest population-based birth cohort of twins ever set up, to study genetic and environmental contributions to weight and eating behaviour during childhood and adolescence. She is also developing interventions that help parents to use feeding practices that support their children in developing healthy eating habits and optimal growth during early life. On a more practical level, she contributes evidence to support UK obesity policy, including how to make obesity public messaging more 'eating-disorders friendly', as part of the Obesity Policy Research Unit. Clare is passionate about science communication; in 2018 she published her book *An Appetite for Life: How to Feed Your Child From the Start*, which offers caregivers advice on how to help their children develop healthy eating habits and a good relationship with food.

JEHANNINE AUSTIN

Jehannine Austin is executive director of the BC Mental Health and Substance Use Services Research Institute, and is a professor in psychiatry and medical genetics at the University of British Columbia. As an undergraduate in biochemistry, they enjoyed studying genetics and decided to do a PhD exploring the genetic variations that make people more vulnerable to developing psychiatric disorders. In retrospect Jehannine recognises one of the contributing factors to this decision was probably their own experience of living with depression and anxiety and their family history of psychiatric illness. Their PhD was very lab based and they felt they didn't have the language to translate their research into concepts that were valuable for people like their family. Jehannine realised there were probably many other families like theirs with similar questions that weren't being answered. This motivated them to become a genetic counsellor so they could learn how to take complex genetic concepts and make it understandable for people in a meaningful way. They were the first person to practise genetic counselling for psychiatric disorders and they have now founded the world's first specialist psychiatric genetic counselling service, which has won an award for its impact on patient outcomes.

5

self-destructive behaviours

INTRODUCTION

Content warning: This chapter discusses self-harm, suicide and other subjects that can be upsetting. Reader discretion is advised.

There are some behaviours that, to someone without first-hand experience, can seem difficult to understand. Many find it difficult to comprehend what motivates people to smoke, take drugs or gamble, for example, and find it easier not to think about shocking acts like suicide and self-harm.

Other examples of self-destructive behaviours tend to remain hidden or disguised. These include self-sabotaging at work or school during times of stress, and deliberately driving away people who care in order to avoid rejection. While to many people these behaviours make little sense, for those affected they feel like important coping mechanisms.

By trying to better understand these different forms of self-destructive behaviours, researchers hope to be able to provide people with alternative, more helpful coping strategies. One problem here is that many people who engage in self-destructive behaviours feel ashamed or guilty about doing so, and this drives them to hide their actions or describe them to healthcare professionals in a certain way because they don't want to cause alarm.

New approaches to research are now providing us with a more realistic estimate of the prevalence of these behaviours, as well as identifying the support services that people are most likely to turn to. Research is also helping in risk assessment by describing the factors that make people more vulnerable to, or more likely to engage in, these behaviours.

This chapter focuses on three forms of self-destructive behaviours: self-harm, addictive behaviours and suicide. These are not mutually exclusive; people often take part in different self-destructive behaviours concurrently or consecutively. These behaviours can, therefore, be risk factors in themselves. For example, self-harm and substance use are considered to be risk factors for suicide. What is key is that in order for someone to give up one of these behaviours, they first need to find other ways of dealing with the difficult thoughts and emotions in their lives.

SELF-HARM

Self-harm refers to any act of intentional self-injury or poisoning, and is used as a means of dealing with feelings, memories or situations that feel painful or overwhelming. There are many ways in which people can self-harm, some more deliberate and direct than others. These include cutting, poisoning, burning, picking or scratching at the skin, hitting oneself or walls, and getting into fights where the person knows they will get hurt.

Self-harm is very complex and the causes and behaviours vary from person to person. For some people self-harm is linked to very specific experiences in the past or present. For others, the cause is less easy to pinpoint and the behaviour may be linked to more general feelings and experiences.

'I realised that, for me, what is difficult about my feelings is they're not tangible or measurable. Through therapy, I've learnt to be much more forgiving of myself and able to accept my emotions, rather than trying to stop them through self-harm.'

EMILY WHEELER

According to mental health charity MIND, self-harm can be a way to:

Express something that is hard to put into words

Turn invisible thoughts or feelings into something visible

Change emotional pain into physical pain

Reduce overwhelming emotional feelings or thoughts

Have a sense of being in control

Escape traumatic memories

Have something in life to rely on

Punish themselves for their feelings and experiences

Stop feeling numb, disconnected or dissociated

Create a reason to physically care for themselves

Express suicidal feelings and thoughts without taking their own life

PROVISION OF SUPPORT

People of all ages and backgrounds engage in self-harm, but it is possible to identify trends in the ways in which people present with self-harm and what happens to them afterwards. This can help to inform policy and practice. Accurate data on self-harm is also crucial in trying to prevent suicide, since a history of self-harm is one of the strongest risk factors associated with suicide.[1]

Around one-quarter of women and one-tenth of men aged between 16 and 24 report having self-harmed in the past.[2] These figures highlight the importance of providing support for those who self-harm when they are young in order to prevent the behaviour from worsening, potentially leading to devastating outcomes.

Research indicates that the occurrence of self-harm is increasing. The reasons for this are unclear, but may relate to a decrease in stigma and improved awareness around mental health. Some trends indicate that alcohol use among young people is decreasing; therefore it may be that some have shifted from one coping mechanism to another.

Clinicians and researchers are concerned that, while the level of awareness around self-harm has improved, the level of support has not increased accordingly. This means that, although young people may feel more able to talk about their behaviour and be receptive to help, that help may not be forthcoming.

In the past, much of the data used to assess levels of self-harm, and inform policy and practice, has come from people either attending an emergency department or being admitted to hospital. More recently, research has looked more widely,[3] and shown that at least half of those who self-harm were not admitted to hospital at all. GP surgeries are an important setting to consider, and research has shown that GPs would welcome more training around self-harm.

Studies show that more males with self-harm (58 per cent) go to an emergency department, but more girls with self-harm access support services in general, and more are admitted overnight to emergency departments. This pattern is particularly clear among 10–15-year-olds (76 per cent of females, compared with 49 per cent of males).[4] These statistics suggest there may be misconceptions around the relative suicide risk for girls and boys, where self-harm in boys is not considered to be as serious as it is in girls. Given the higher overall suicide rate in males, emergency departments may be important as a setting when looking to improve the support provided to young men who self-harm.

There is also concern over a lack of consistency in how ambulance services care for patients who have self-harmed[5] and how or if they are referred to mental health services. Research shows that ambulance staff would like more training and education around self-harm.

FLUIDITY AND RISK ASSESSMENT

Self-harm is not always a constant or consistent behaviour. Someone's vulnerability to it can change over time, as can the level and type of self-harm that they engage in. There isn't a threshold that needs to be passed for someone to self-harm and triggers can vary. What's more, although self-harm is a risk factor for suicide, the two are not inevitably linked. All of this makes it difficult to assess the risk of self-harm at any one point in time.

It's important to understand that self-harming behaviour means different things to people at different times in their lives. It offers them different coping strategies for different feelings. Having self-harmed, people often feel a sense of short-term release, but the effects can diminish over time, meaning feelings of self-worth, hopelessness and punishment return. Assessing what self-harm means for people may be more important than describing the details of what they do. It may also give us more of an insight into what is likely to happen over time.

Although awareness around the existence of self-harm has improved in recent years, it is still a topic that is often met with shock and fear. As well as being hurtful for the person who is self-harming, this reaction can close down potentially helpful discussions. To find new ways of talking about self-harm and to better understand its complexity, researchers have developed the Card Sort Task for Self-Harm (CaTS).[6] Here, patients are given cards that are categorised into broad groups of thoughts, feelings, events, behaviour, self-harm support and services, and asked to place them along a timeline, starting from six months before self-harm. This process has been shown to be particularly powerful in helping young people to visualise the sequence of events over time and broach difficult subjects in a non-verbal way.

Researchers are further co-developing the CaTS approach with young people so that it might be used as a clinical tool for assessment and support and eventually be available in digital format or as an app.

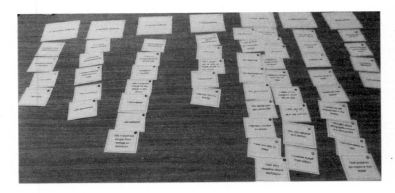

'The cards give people permission to say what has happened to them. You might not be able to talk about it, but you can put a card down to represent your self-harm. People find that quite powerful and often when they work with the cards they have these lightbulb moments where they realise what the transitions were that moved them towards a behaviour and what might move them away from it.'

PROFESSOR ELLEN TOWNSEND

RISK FACTORS FOR SELF-HARM

Research shows that an important factor in the development of self-harming behaviours is loneliness.[7] Being alone can amplify feelings of depression and worry and compound the person's sense of having no one to talk to or to understand their need to self-harm.

Given that during the Covid-19 pandemic many people felt more lonely than usual, one might have expected levels of self-harm to increase. However, a review of research in this area shows there were, in fact, fewer people presenting to services with self-harm in the first half of 2021.[8] Researchers have suggested that the reduction in numbers may be down to people seeking less help during the pandemic, or finding alternative sources of support when social distancing measures were in place. This demonstrates how variations in situations and the environment can influence risk factors for self-harm.

Researchers have also investigated how different aspects of neurodiversity and school behaviour may relate to self-harm in young people. One study showed that the risk of self-harm (in terms of presenting to hospital emergency departments) was nearly three times higher for boys with autism spectrum disorder (ASD) than those without the condition.[9] This pattern was not seen in girls. ADHD and absence from school were also strong predictors of self-harm, for both boys and girls.

As well as individual factors that may place people at risk of self-harm, it's important to identify the places where at-risk young people tend to present. Young Offender Institutions, pupil referral units, children's homes, and other services catering for young people who have been excluded from mainstream education and care are all settings where vulnerability to self-harm may be high.

SMARTPHONE USE AND SOCIAL MEDIA

A major influence on young people and their likelihood of self-harming is social media. According to research, many young people are showing a form of addictive behaviour where they feel anxious if they cannot check their smartphones.[10] Studies have also found a link between people watching or seeing content that involves self-harm and those individuals self-harming or having thoughts of suicide themselves.[11] Greater time spent on online social networking promotes self-harm behaviour and suicidal ideation in vulnerable adolescents.[12]

Although research has shown patterns between social media, smartphone use and self-harm, there is still a gap in our knowledge about how it actually impacts on mental health and self-harm. This gap needs to be bridged in order that we might be able to help young people maintain the benefits of social media and smartphone use without experiencing negative effects.

One project is working with young people who have accessed mental health services to try to understand these links better.[13] The study aims to learn when and what type of support would be useful for young people who are experiencing difficulties. Still more research is needed in this area, not only to help young people, but also to inform regulation on social media platforms.

TAKING RESPONSIBILITY ACROSS SOCIETY

There remain challenges to researching self-harm, which means there are still many unknowns around its prevalence and how best to support those who are self-harming. Among these challenges is the reluctance of those in primary and secondary care to record self-harm because of concerns around labelling people or having to decide what to do next. Healthcare and other professionals often record and treat the physical symptoms (cutting, bruising etc.) without considering it to be self-harm, meaning the underlying causes go unaddressed.

There is a need, therefore, to open up conversations around self-harm in healthcare services, as well as in schools, workplaces, and social and legal systems. Self-harm is the responsibility not just of mental healthcare professionals, but a range of services. To enable this sense of broader responsibility, people need to feel they are informed, but also that there are actions they can take to provide support. There is also a need to improve training and support.

One of the most-used clinical research tools in mental health is a questionnaire called the PHQ-9, which provides information on a range of mental health conditions. This does include a question on self-harm, but it tends to be removed when used in research projects, because researchers who receive information about participants self-harming might have to break confidentiality. Unfortunately, it means that many research projects looking at mental health could be missing important information on self-harm.

It should be remembered that there are also certain groups of people who are vulnerable to self-harm, but who as a result of their actions are often viewed unsympathetically in society's eyes. These people may be harming others through bullying or fighting, they may be drinking or using drugs, they may be homeless or judged as manipulative and attention-seeking. This link tends to compound even further the societal fear and stigma that surrounds self-harm.

The ongoing development of research using electronic records and cross-referencing sets of data from health, education and legal systems is enabling hidden behaviours such as these to surface, and voices that might otherwise have gone unnoticed to be heard. However, this needs to happen within an informed and accepting society, so that the right preventative and supportive work can be done at scale.

'*Even though research shows how common self-harm is, there is still a reluctance to accept this and to support young people. In an average class of thirty 14-year-olds, there will be at least three who are self-harming. These young people are supporting each other and talking about it but often the adults around them step away from the subject and from starting conversations that could help their understanding.*'

PROFESSOR ANN JOHN

'There is still a lot of stigma around self-harm and, unfortunately, it stops people from seeking help and from understanding what's happening or responding appropriately. When you want to ask questions or do some work around self-harm people get very nervous. I think, in part, that stems from the idea that if you ask about self-harm it will plant the idea and make it more common, but there's no evidence that this is the case.'

PROFESSOR ANN JOHN

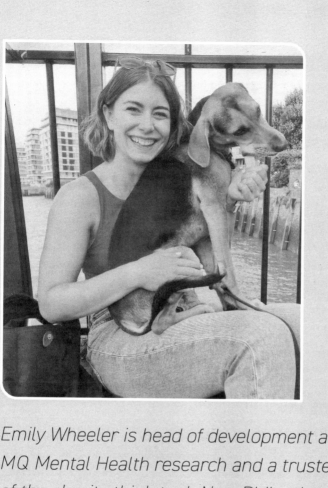

Emily Wheeler is head of development at MQ Mental Health research and a trustee of the charity think tank New Philanthropy Capital (NPC), and until mid-2022 was the chair of Nightline Association, the umbrella organisation that supports Nightlines, peer-to-peer listening support services for 1.6 million students across the UK.

It's difficult to know exactly when it started. I think my brain has blocked out the memories. I had a very happy childhood and a very stable family but when I was a teenager, I started having these feelings of what I now know to be anxiety. I had a lot of self-doubt and self-hate, and my head just wasn't a very nice place to be.

I started to get this very physical feeling that was a tightness in my chest. It mostly happened when I went to bed and when I was alone with my own thoughts. And somehow my brain made this connection between this very physical feeling and a physical way to get rid of it.

I think it started with whacking my head against a wall and then it escalated into worse ways to alleviate this feeling. For me that was cutting – on my arms and legs – in places that couldn't be seen. It was like an addiction because the cutting got worse and worse so I could get the same effect. But in the end it didn't help; if anything, it would make it and the feelings of guilt worse.

HIDING AND GUILT

I hid it from everyone. I never went to A&E. Even in warm weather I would wear long sleeves and fingerless gloves. On the outside I was bubbly and happy. I was doing really well at school, I had lots of friends and I had partners over the years. Nothing would suggest there was anything else going on.

Then one day I got out of the shower and my sister saw the cuts on my leg. At that stage I didn't know how to explain it and the thought of my family knowing about my self-harm made it even worse because I felt so guilty. So I tried to stop the self-harm, but during that time I started to experience what I now know are panic attacks. Often I would be getting ready to go to school and a few things would go wrong and I would get that physical tightness in my chest and it was just too much – as I couldn't self-harm to cope, I'd break down, cry, shout and take it out on those closest to me, like my mum.

And that was what my mum saw – mood swings – and that was why she ended up taking me to the doctor's. The doctor took a blood test, looking for low sugar levels, but when they came back clear they told me I was fine and off they sent me with just the explanation of it being normal teenage behaviour.

FLUCTUATIONS

At some point the self-harm just seemed to fade out of my life. Again, I don't have clear memories of when it stopped. Then in my second year at university a lot of things happened at once: the deaths of my grandparents, exams and deadlines. Self-harm didn't cross my mind but one day, towards the end of a seminar, I started feeling sick and dizzy. I decided to go to the doctor's and when I got there I just burst into tears and was having a full-on panic attack. More followed that year and luckily my tutors were really supportive with extended deadlines, but, again, I never sought or was offered medical help.

Post-university and in work, it was almost like all of that was behind me. I was still very hard on myself but self-harm and panic attacks felt like a thing of the past, something from my difficult teenage phase. However, it was in my mid-twenties when suddenly it felt like I was stuck in the role I was in, I wasn't progressing and I wasn't achieving and suddenly I started feeling more anxious. I started having the feelings of a panic attack bubbling up and having to run out of the office and just get into the fresh air. Then the thoughts of self-harm started creeping back in, like intrusive thoughts, so bad on a few occasions I called Samaritans, needing someone to help me calm down and stop me from acting on them. The thoughts were so intrusive and I couldn't stop them and a few times I lost that battle with myself and would end up self-harming. Alcohol also played a role for me. It was like when I'd had something to drink, the thoughts more easily entered my mind and my rational side didn't have as much control to stop myself acting on them. I couldn't believe I was back here again. I tried to seek medical support but with long waiting lists I never got the help I needed.

LEARNING TO SIT WITH FEELINGS

Changing jobs and finding one where I felt fulfilled helped me again move through this period. So it wasn't until I was about 26 or 27 that I first went to therapy. At the time things were going well but I thought it would be a good time to try some preventative work. With the first person I saw the relationship was really uncomfortable. I am lucky that I'd been working in mental health in my new job so I knew it might take a while to find the right person and was in a good enough place where I had the energy, and the finances, to persevere. So I stopped and found someone else. And she was fantastic. It was just the right fit. I started to understand my self-harm – not just the triggers but the patterns of thinking that were behind it. And it allowed me to actually talk about self-harm openly, which was so important.

Through this process, I realised that for me one of the difficulties with feelings is that they're not tangible or measurable, but through therapy I have learnt to be much more forgiving on myself and to be able to accept my emotions rather than trying to stop them through self-harm. I understand now that it's OK to feel upset, rather than tell myself I shouldn't be feeling that and beat myself up. I also realised that self-harm and anxiety will always be a part of my make-up, from the scars through to the way I think, and that these intrusive thoughts can come back. I don't always win the battle but now I have the tools that mean I win most of the time.

POSSIBLE PREVENTION

I think the school environment is really important as a place to provide information and support, particularly around it being OK to feel different feelings, and it needs to happen at an early age and with the support of parents. Essentially, we're playing catch-up with a whole generation of people who didn't have this kind of information and support and I think a wider approach could really help to lessen the fear around self-harm.

And once we have that awareness, we need to make sure that young people have the coping mechanisms so they don't have to resort to self-harm. For me self-harm was a coping mechanism. It didn't work, it made it worse, but it was my attempt at finding a way to lessen these horrible feelings. Maybe if I had been taught a better coping mechanism then the self-harm never would have happened.

TACKLING FEAR WITH RESEARCH

People get very scared when they think about self-harm. I have had moments where I have felt suicidal but again, I'm lucky that I've never got to the stage where I've made a plan. So for me, I see the two as linked, but they can also be separate and I think a lot of people don't necessarily see that. I know it's hard because self-harm can be a risk factor, but because it is so often attached to suicide it makes people even more scared to talk about it.

To me this is where research is so important: to enable people to understand this big scary thing out there that is mental illness in all of its colours. Research can deliver the tools to help us with mental health and without research, it's just guesswork. We need to understand self-harm to help people find a coping mechanism that works for them and helps them live happier, healthier and more fulfilling lives.

ADDICTIVE BEHAVIOURS

Addiction covers a wide range of behaviours and does not relate only to drugs and alcohol. It includes behaviours such as gambling, overeating, sex, exercise, playing video games, love, internet use, social media use and work. It affects people of all ages and, as with other self-destructive behaviours, it is surrounded by various myths and preconceptions.

The word 'addict' tends to have negative connotations and is often used to describe everyday behaviour around people's relationship to activities and objects. There is a continuum in addictive behaviour, and whether it is considered to be problematic relates to the extent of its negative impacts and withdrawal effects on day-to-day life. A subjective sense of losing control is also considered part of addictive behaviour.

The key element of an addiction is that the person is not able to control their behaviour as they would like and their behaviour can become extreme, affecting their day-to-day functioning. It has been argued that people can become addicted to almost anything if the behaviour provides constant rewards;[14] however, the overarching definition of addiction is that it is a repetitive habit pattern that increases the risk of disease and/or personal and social problems. The challenges in changing an addictive behaviour (via treatment or self-initiation) are also typical features of its definition.

COMPONENTS OF ADDICTION

Although diverse in nature, addictive behaviours have elements in common and these reflect, in part, the clinical criteria for addiction. Researchers have conceptualised addictions in terms of these similarities and developed the 'components model of addiction'.[15] This proposes that all genuine addictive behaviours have six core components (see below) and when people behave in a way that fulfils these six they can be defined as being addicted to that behaviour.

Salience: This refers to how important the behaviour is to the individual. Addictive behaviours become the most important activity for a person, so that even when they are not doing it, they are thinking about it. There is also 'reverse salience', which is when they are prevented from engaging in the behaviour and it becomes all they can think about. One example might be a smoker on a long-haul flight.

Mood modification: This is the experience that people report having when carrying out their addictive behaviour. People with addictive behaviour patterns commonly report a 'rush', 'buzz' or 'high', for example, when they take drugs or are gambling. What is interesting is that a person's drug or activity of choice can have the capacity to achieve different mood-modifying effects at different times; sometimes it can be a rush and at other times a relaxant.

Tolerance: This refers to the increasing amount of activity that is required to achieve the same effect. The classic example of tolerance is a heroin addict's need to increase the size of their 'fix' to get the type of feeling they once got from much smaller doses. In gambling, tolerance may involve the gambler gradually having to increase the size of the bet or spending longer periods gambling.

Withdrawal symptoms: These are the unpleasant feelings and physical effects that occur when the addictive behaviour is suddenly discontinued or reduced. They can include 'the shakes', moodiness and irritability. These symptoms are commonly believed to be a response to the removal of a chemical that the person has become dependent on. However, these effects can also be experienced by gamblers, so the effects may be due to withdrawal from the behaviour as well as the substance.

Conflict: People with addictive behaviours develop conflicts with the people around them, as well as within themselves. Continual choosing of short-term pleasure and relief leads to disregard of adverse consequences and long-term damage, which in turn increases the apparent need for the addictive activity as a coping strategy. The person knows they are engaging too much in the behaviour and tries to cut down or stop. However, they feel unable to do so and experience a subjective loss of control.

Relapse: This refers to the tendency towards repeated reversions to earlier patterns of the particular activity. Even the most extreme patterns typical of the height of the addiction can be quickly restored after many years of abstinence or control. Such relapses are common in all addictions, including behavioural addictions such as gambling.

MODELS OF ADDICTIVE BEHAVIOUR

The model that we use to explain addiction affects how we view the person with the addictive behaviour and also how we decide to 'treat' their behaviour in order to change it. There are numerous models of addictive behaviour and, although there are clear differences between the theories, they overlap and can contribute to our understanding of the complexities of addictions.

Interestingly, the theories appear to vary in the amount of control they attribute to the individual, with more biological explanations often suggesting the individual is biologically destined to take a path of addiction. The more environmental explanations suggest that the influences on addiction are numerous and varied, and that individuals may exert more choice over their behaviours through their environment and surroundings.

MODELS OF ADDICTIVE BEHAVIOUR

The disease model suggests that addiction comes from a disorder of the body, such as a chemical imbalance in the brain. In this model, the individual has limited control over their behaviour in the same way that a person has limited control over whether or not they catch an infectious disease.

The genetic model suggests there is a genetic disposition towards addictive behaviour. The influence of genes and environment can be difficult to unpick. For example, the biggest risk factor for becoming a cigarette smoker is having parents who smoke, but does this show evidence of a genetic disposition or family influence? With advances in genetic analysis and databases, research is now showing a higher incidence of specific genes in people with addictive behaviours.

The experiential model suggests that addictive behaviours are much more temporary and dependent on the situation we are in than either of the previous two models. In fact, people often move on from (or grow out of) their addictive behaviours as their life circumstances change.

The moral model suggests that the key issue with addiction is a lack of character. In this view, addiction is a result of weakness or moral failure in the individual. The treatment for this is to get people to repent and then to develop their moral strength.

The biological model focuses on the role of chemicals in the brain, and on genetic differences between people with and without addictions. This fits better with chemical addictions, such as nicotine and drugs, than behaviours such as gambling.

In biological models, the susceptibility (whether genetic or neurochemical) is most likely to take effect during the time when the behaviour starts, rather than the period when it is maintained. However, if a person does manage to give up their addiction, this biological predisposition would make the person more vulnerable to becoming addicted again.

BRAIN CHEMISTRY

A neurotransmitter is a chemical that moves between nerve cells to transmit messages, and the one that is most commonly connected to addiction is dopamine. Dopamine plays a major role in the brain's reward system and has been linked with the rewarding effects of substances and alcohol.

The brain's reward system is influential in how we learn, because we tend to repeat behaviours that are rewarded. From an evolutionary perspective, this brain reward enhanced our chances of survival by giving priority to beneficial actions such as reproduction. Certain substances are able to influence the brain reward pathway, either by directly influencing the action of dopamine or by altering the activity of other chemicals that influence this pathway, such as GABA, serotonin and opioids. As well as playing a role in chemical addictions, neurotransmitters have been implicated in behaviours such as gambling[16] and video game playing.[17]

The complex effects of neurotransmitters are not fully understood; it is difficult to identify which neurotransmitter produces which reward, and the effects of one drug can be very diverse. For example, research has shown that nicotine can affect several systems simultaneously, including learning and memory, the control of pain and the relief of anxiety.[18] It is generally believed that smoking nicotine increases arousal and reduces stress, two responses often considered to be incompatible. This means it is difficult to pin down a single response that follows smoking a cigarette, taking a drug or engaging in an addictive behaviour. Research is increasingly demonstrating that there are multiple neurotransmitter systems (e.g. dopaminergic, serotonergic) involved in gambling disorders.[19]

GENETICS OF ADDICTION

How the reward system in the brain functions is affected by genetic and environmental factors. Historically, we have investigated genetic factors in human behaviour by studying family relationships, particularly by comparing identical and non-identical twins. It is now possible also to analyse the genes themselves and look for differences in the genetic structure of people with and without addictive behaviours.[20]

Family studies tend to emphasise the role of environmental factors in the development of addictive behaviours. A study of over 300 identical twins and just under 200 same-sex non-identical twins showed that the major influences on the decision to use substances were environmental rather than genetic.[21]

Studies also indicate a link between genetics and personality traits in addictive behaviours. For example, a study of identical and non-identical twins showed a connection between genetics and antisocial personality characteristics (such as attention seeking, not following social norms and violence), and between these personality characteristics and alcoholism.[22] There have been similar findings for behavioural addictions such as gambling.[23]

Over the years, scientists have identified multiple genes linked to addictive behaviours, but one single gene has not been found to be responsible. Several genes have been implicated in alcoholism, and others linked to addiction to cannabis and cocaine. Genetic studies examining problem gambling have noted that genes involved in the dopamine and serotonin systems may increase vulnerability to developing a gambling disorder.[24]

Increasingly, the evidence suggests that environmental factors such as stress can influence so-called epigenetic changes, which can trigger the development of addiction. Epigenetic changes do not involve changes in the actual sequence of the genetic material (DNA), but instead change how the gene takes action to influence behaviour and characteristics. One of the systems that is affected by stress hormones is the brain's reward circuitry and it is proposed that this could be partly through epigenetic changes.

Explanations that revolve around brain chemicals and genetics help to account for inherent vulnerabilities and susceptibilities when people first become addicted. They also provide a reason as to why some people may be more resistant to addiction treatment and more prone to returning to addictions, even when they have managed to stop. However, they can't explain everything about addiction and the social and cultural contexts in which these behaviours occur need to be considered.

ADDICTION AND AVAILABILITY

A number of environmental factors affect the level, severity and impact of addictive behaviours in a society. For example, the level of alcoholism is influenced by the availability and average consumption of alcohol by the general population. Studies comparing the number of deaths through liver cirrhosis (generally attributed to alcohol abuse) around the world have found a strong link with the average consumption of alcohol in those countries.[25]

The so-called 'availability factor' also affects gambling. For instance, in a study of five US states[26] harmful gambling was found to have increased after a rise in the accessibility of gambling. Elsewhere, a study[27] found that the level of problem gambling was proportional to the length of time that had elapsed since the new gambling opportunities had been available to the public. Despite evidence pointing to a link between gambling and accessibility, however, we cannot establish that accessibility is the cause. It is important to consider also the potential impact of public initiatives aimed at tackling gambling, such as awareness campaigns, helplines and professional counselling programmes. These initiatives most likely alter the relationship between increased opportunities to gamble and problem gambling.

COGNITIVE EXPLANATIONS OF ADDICTIVE BEHAVIOUR

Exploring thinking processes and biases is particularly helpful in understanding behavioural addictions such as gambling. Compared with biological models, cognitive models of addictive behaviour tend to focus more on the maintenance phase and thought patterns, or biases, around the addictive behaviour, which keep it going and make people more susceptible to relapse should they give up.

In gambling, for example, the odds are weighted strongly in favour of the gambling operator, yet gamblers continue to believe they can win money. This suggests that gambling may be maintained by beliefs that are wrong or irrational.[28] People tend to overestimate the extent to which they can predict or influence gambling outcomes and misjudge how much money they have won or lost.[29]

BEHAVIOURAL EXPLANATIONS OF ADDICTIVE BEHAVIOUR

The basis of behavioural theories is the idea of learning and conditioning, whereby a particular stimulus or signal becomes increasingly effective in evoking a response. For instance, a drug addict might experience a craving for heroin at the sight of a hypodermic needle, while a gambling addict might get a strong craving to gamble if they walk past a bookmaker's.

Addicts may also change their behaviour in response to rewards and punishments, so when an alcoholic drinks it might give them pleasure or relieve withdrawal symptoms. These rewards and punishments can bring about changes in mood or something more material, such as money, which then impacts on behaviour. Interestingly, research on animals has found that a greater behavioural change was achieved by a lower level of reinforcement, an effect further strengthened when the arrival of these reinforcements was less predictable. This has implications for why addicts may continue certain behaviours even when they don't produce rewards or positive effects every time. It may be that it is not just the reward itself, but the expectation of reward that is important.

PERSONALITY AND ADDICTION

Psychological research into why some individuals are more prone to addictions suggests that addicts share many characteristics. For instance, research following children through to adulthood has shown that adolescents who are 'rebellious' and have 'less conventional attitudes' are more likely to abuse alcohol, nicotine and illicit drugs.[30]

The term 'addictive personality' has become widespread in its usage and suggests that some people are more prone to addiction than others as a result of their personalities. However, there is no personality trait that is predictive of addiction and addiction alone.[31] The role of personality in addiction is unclear and it is difficult to disentangle the effects of personality on addiction from the effects of addiction on personality. To determine that there is an addictive personality, standards of proof would need to be met, including demonstrating that the trait exists before the addiction develops and that the trait is specific to the addiction.[32]

TREATMENTS AND THERAPIES

Cognitive behavioural therapy provides one way to address the patterns in thinking and behaviour that are central to any addiction. Addiction often involves conflicted behaviour, where people engage in behaviours or use substances despite knowing the risks and consequences. CBT helps the person to examine their thoughts, feelings and triggers, and develop different thinking patterns that lead to alternative behaviours. As addiction often starts as a way of coping with difficult feelings and situations, CBT also teaches new coping skills, including for cravings and relapses.

Medication is used to help re-establish normal brain function and decrease cravings in opioid (heroin, prescription pain relievers), tobacco (nicotine) and alcohol addiction. For heroin addiction, morphine, methadone and buprenorphine act on the same receptors in the brain as heroin but suppress withdrawal symptoms and relieve cravings. Other medications are in development to treat stimulant (cocaine, methamphetamine) and cannabis (marijuana) addiction.

Nicotine replacement therapies, available in various forms, are used for addiction to smoking, and vaping has also become a popular alternative. Research into vaping is still in its infancy.

DETOXIFICATION

The aim of detox is to enable a safe and humane withdrawal from addiction and to prepare the person for ongoing treatment. Some detoxification procedures are specific to particular drugs, while others are based on general principles of treatment. Before starting detox, an initial medical assessment evaluates the likely severity of withdrawal alongside any other physical and mental health conditions. While medication is often used to help with withdrawal, it is not the only component of treatment. Psychological support is also important in reducing the patient's distress during detoxification.

REDUCING HARM

Harm reduction refers to interventions aimed at reducing the negative effects of health behaviours, without necessarily extinguishing them completely. Most research and initiatives in this area focus on drug addiction, with strategies including provision of clean syringes, testing for hepatitis or HIV, overdose prevention and reversal, drug consumption rooms and information on safer drug use. It is, however, an approach that has also been applied to other harmful behaviours, such as sex work and eating disorders.

As a philosophy, harm reduction is grounded in justice and human rights, and focuses on working with people without judgement, coercion, discrimination, or the requirement that they stop their addictive behaviours.

Taken on their own, the different models – biological, cognitive, behavioural or personality – face challenges in providing a complete explanation for addictive behaviour. To account for the full diversity of addictive patterns and behaviour, we need to consider different elements from these theories.

Research and practices aiming at helping those with addictions are best served by an approach that incorporates the best strands of contemporary psychology, biology and sociology. This eclectic perspective provides the most all-encompassing view of addictive behaviour.

TAKE-HOME NALOXONE

Globally, about 150,000 people die each year from drug overdoses, and this is despite an antidote to the effects of opioids, called naloxone, saving lives in hospitals and in the hands of paramedics. In most cases of overdoses, however, the emergency services cannot reach the person immediately. One solution, take-home naloxone (THN), has now been implemented in 23 countries, enabling the antidote to be administered by non-medics where and when it is required. Research is ongoing to make it more available, acceptable and effective. This may include developing a nasal spray to avoid administration via injection.

FOCUS ON RECOVERY

Despite the importance of recovery in helping those with addictions, there has been little consensus on what recovery really means or how to assess it. The Substance Use Recovery Evaluator (SURE)[33] was developed to provide some level of common understanding around the concept of recovery. Aimed at use with alcohol and drug addiction, it consists of 21 questions that measure five key dimensions of recovery: alcohol and other drug use; self-care; relationships; material resources; and outlook on life. Available as an app and a dashboard, this tool gives people a means of identifying personal goals.

THINKING PATTERNS OF GAMBLERS

Researchers have investigated whether people who gamble regularly think and behave differently to non-regular gamblers by identifying and comparing how they talk about and explain their gambling and its outcomes.[34] Gamblers were found to use more irrational descriptions and explanations and to personify the gambling machine: 'The machine hates me' or 'This fruity is in a good mood'. They also tended to explain their losses in terms of hindsight and previous predictions: 'I had a feeling it wasn't going to pay', 'I had a feeling it was going to chew up those tokens', etc.

Interestingly, irrational thought processes don't appear to be linked to other aspects of gambling, such as risk-taking or how many times a behaviour is rewarded. It may be, therefore, that these irrational thought processes don't drive gambling, but result from the challenge of trying to come up with meaningful statements in situations that are essentially determined by chance. This makes it difficult to establish cause and effect of cognitive biases.

'Some individuals engage in behaviours that have addictive elements without it being a full-blown addiction. This raises questions. For example, if someone has no negative withdrawal effects after stopping cocaine use or gambling, are they addicted? If the cocaine use or gambling does not conflict with anything else in that person's life, can it be said to be an addiction? In very simple terms, the difference between an excessive enthusiasm and an addiction is that enthusiasm adds to life whereas addiction takes away from it.'

PROFESSOR MARK GRIFFITHS

'The experience of pleasure is very important for our healthy development. If, for example, we found food or sex boring, then our species would probably have failed. The feelings of pleasure associated with these activities act as a reinforcement. If we associate them with other activities, then they too will be reinforced. The pleasure that encourages essential behaviours is therefore also the pleasure that can encourage damaging behaviour. Could it be that the threat of addiction is the price we pay for pleasure?'

PROFESSOR MARK GRIFFITHS

'Just because a person has some of the personality traits of addiction does not mean they are, or will become, an addict. Practitioners consider specific traits to be warning signs (e.g. neuroticism), but that's all they are. No personality trait guarantees addiction. In short, there is little evidence for an addictive personality as such.'

PROFESSOR MARK GRIFFITHS

'Addiction is a multifaceted behaviour that is strongly influenced by contextual factors, and these cannot be encompassed by any single theoretical perspective. These factors include variations in behavioural involvement and motivation across different demographic groups, structural characteristics of activities/substances, and the developmental or temporal nature of addictive behaviour.'

PROFESSOR MARK GRIFFITHS

SPOTLIGHT: ADDICTION TO GAMBLING

Gambling is a relatively new member of those behaviours considered to be an addiction. It is acceptable and legal in most countries but has always been considered clandestine and confined to certain locations. Awareness and openness around gambling is increasing, but it faces the same stigma as other addictions.

THE THINKING AROUND GAMBLING: SKILLS AND CHANCE

One valuable explanation for problem gambling and gambling addictions lies in the role of thoughts, beliefs and attitudes. Many factors may play a role in the acquisition, development and maintenance of gambling addiction, among them personality traits, biological processes, unconscious motivations and learning, as well as idiosyncratic factors, such as financial motivation and economic pressures.

Many of the thought processes that researchers believe underlie gambling behaviour are more likely when an activity is perceived to have a level of skill.[35] Indeed, there is a genuine possibility for skilful play and improvement in games such as blackjack and poker, and in sports betting. This means that beliefs about control and skill are neither completely irrational nor consistent across gamblers.

Even in activities where outcomes are chance-determined, there are likely to be variations in the extent to which gamblers perceive that the outcomes are down to luck. Those activities or games with more complex rules and a greater number of playing strategies are, for example, more likely to be perceived as skilful. This means behavioural addictions like gambling tend to be very varied and have a large subjective element.

GETTING HOOKED

Learning principles have been applied to the study of gambling. One theory proposes that problem gambling and persistent gambling are maintained by reward in terms of the money won.[36] The rewards are not constant or predictable, which explains why people keep gambling in the hope that next time they will win.

Activities such as slot machines and scratchcards, where there is a short time interval between stake and outcome, and where outcomes are entirely determined by chance, appear to fit this explanation better than others. In skilled gambling games, such as blackjack, poker and sports betting, the gambler's decisions can influence outcomes significantly, so it is more difficult to apply the same principles. There are also questions over how well this theory explains excessive gambling, where gamblers typically lose more than they win and where the rewards are dependent on gambler responses, such as stake sizes.[37]

Another approach, classical conditioning, suggests that individuals continue to gamble as a result of the excitement or arousal associated with it, and that they feel bored, unstimulated and restless when they are not gambling. This provides a better explanation of people's motivation to start a gambling session and why they become excessive gamblers, but appears less useful in explaining why people continue to gamble.

IMPORTANCE OF CONTEXT

Environmental and circumstantial factors are also central to understanding gambling addiction, and often facilitate and encourage people to gamble in the first place.[38] The location of the venue, number of venues in a specified area and possible membership requirements can affect how accessible or easy it is to gamble.

Even internal features of the venue, such as the decor, heating, lighting, background music, layout, refreshment facilities and the placement of the cash dispenser can be influential. Other motivational factors include advertising, free travel and/or accommodation to the gambling venue, free bets or gambles on particular games, and availability of free food and/or alcoholic drinks while gambling.

Structural characteristics, built into the game or gambling structure, can also be important in the development of addictive behaviour.[39] Examples of these are seen in slot machines, where the game speed is fast and there are large jackpots, lots of 'near misses' and short payout intervals. These features are specifically designed to keep people gambling once they have started.

THE ADDICTIVE POWER OF SLOT MACHINES

Research has shown that gambling activities characterised by short-event frequencies, such as slot machines, are the ones most played by problem gamblers. Many slot machine players overestimate the amount of skill involved when playing such games. When combined with motivational factors (e.g. gambling as a way of escape), slot machine gamblers may become conditioned to the 'tranquillising' effect of engaging in the activity, rather than the simple desire to win money. The fast speed of play in these high-event-frequency activities has been linked to problem gambling, as have continuous forms of gambling (e.g. casino games, in-play sports betting, slot machines) with rapid play rates.

'In the case of gambling, biological and psychological factors are not the only major sets of influences. Different structural characteristics (e.g. event frequency, near misses) may have implications for the gambler's motivations and, as a consequence, the social impact of gambling.'

PROFESSOR MARK GRIFFITHS

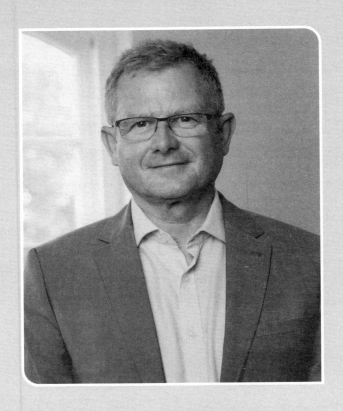

Peter Higgins is a 56-year-old gambling addict who began his gambling at the age of 17 and has finally stopped (fingers crossed, as he says himself). He has been a functioning addict, actually working within the gambling industry for most of his working life, with some of the largest digital bookmaking firms as well as running his own small bookmaking

business (shop, phone and online). Currently he acts as a mediator, predominantly in the commercial sector and often with the gambling industry. He has simultaneously embarked upon a masters degree in 'addiction psychology and counselling' with a view to qualifying as a counsellor enabling him to work with addicts. He feels that his own lived experience, allied to a deeper understanding of the theoretical aspects of addiction, could provide those addicted with a useful combination that may help them through their addiction.

I was 17 years old when I had my first bet. I won, but looking back I can see it was one of the worst days of my life.

I was working at a football club when one of the players asked me if I wanted to come and put a bet on a horse they'd been tipped off on. I was earning £25 a week and bet £10 of it, but the horse won and I doubled my earnings in seconds. It was my first bet and I was with the others, and it was this euphoric moment. The same day, I went to the greyhound track with a friend and I won £200 in a few hours.

From then on, I started to place small bets, but over time I needed to do more and more to achieve the same buzz. When it came to betting, my sense of value would go and I'd throw away money without thinking. It's like I was immersed in a different world, a very isolated one.

RECOGNISING THE PROBLEM

In the initial stages, I knew I had an addiction problem, but brushed it off. However, it was the first thing I thought about in the morning and started to take up every moment of my life. I played football for the local team, and even on the journey there and while playing I'd be thinking about betting.

Then online betting came on the scene. In the early days, it wasn't regulated and you could bet on anything, at any time. I didn't need to know the teams or the form; often I wasn't even watching the game or the race. I'd skip meeting up with friends so I could put bets on and started lying to cover it up. When I did go out socially, I would get agitated because I couldn't put a bet on and I was imagining what had happened.

Gambling is the most private disease out there. There's no giveaway sign.

STAGES OF STOPPING

In the end, I created my own betting brand, trying to flip from being punter to bookie. I got a buzz from people losing their bets, rather than from me winning. In some ways it was a sensible approach to stopping, but it didn't work, nor did trying to find something to replace the buzz. I tried to go cold turkey and lasted two weekends, which felt like two years. On the third weekend I allowed myself one small bet. I justified it and rationalised it, but it didn't work.

In the end, it was a combination of having children and embarrassment that stopped me. I wasn't happy with who I was and what I was doing. I didn't like being deceitful and hiding things. What made the big difference was really wanting to manage my urges to bet, because previously I didn't. Something flipped, so I felt increasingly proud when I didn't place a bet. The feeling of control came to outweigh the buzz of winning.

HELPING OTHERS

Addicts need to find their own way to achieve that control; some may do it in three weeks, others may never manage it. It took me 15 years. I'd like to see more harm reduction, so that instead of being told they have to abstain, people might be able to partake in gambling in a safe environment.

SUICIDE

Researchers and clinicians often describe the devastating impact of suicide as a set of ripples, because of the number of lives touched. Suicide is the second most common cause of death in young people worldwide and it has been estimated that for every death by suicide around 135 people will be affected.[40]

Suicide is still a taboo subject, one that we don't want to think about or talk about, and that we fear. But it is by bringing suicide into our discussions and conversations that we can support those considering suicide and make a change. Research can help unveil the subject, dispelling myths that surround it and contributing to the development of new approaches to help reduce the numbers of people who die by suicide.

According to the WHO, there are about 703,000 suicides, globally, each year. Every 40 seconds one person dies from suicide and 20 people will attempt suicide. The numbers are shocking and, yet, in statistical terms, suicide is a rare event, and therefore difficult to predict or anticipate. To add to the challenge, as with self-harm suicide risk is very dynamic by nature. It can fluctuate daily and even hourly, depending on what is happening in that person's life and in their environment.

Research into the risk of suicide in people with depression that took place between 2007 and 2017 showed one in every 1,000 reported considering suicide and one in every 2,000 were at high risk of suicide. These numbers increased over the ten-year period.

Although risk of suicide is closely linked to mental health conditions, in the UK only a third of those who die by suicide are in contact with mental health services in the year before they die. This compares to 80 per cent who are in contact with primary healthcare services.[41] This demonstrates the importance of building awareness around suicide in all services, with particular consideration of the most common points of contact for people considering suicide. People who die by suicide may not present to services with suicidal thinking or ideation, but rather with a range of other behaviours, such as depression, long-term health conditions and substance use.

PREVALENCE AND RESEARCH

Although we have figures at a global and national level for suicide occurrence, it is thought that these are underestimates. New approaches are using electronic health records to provide more accurate estimates and to improve our understanding of how a person goes from thinking about suicide to acting on those thoughts.

Studies are developing models of risk prediction in real time, considering factors such as substance abuse, psychiatric disorders, injury and chronic conditions.[42, 43] Researchers are also looking at how to combine data from health records and from brief self-report questionnaires collected at emergency departments to improve the strength of prediction.[44]

Novel approaches using natural language processing (NLP) are enabling the analysis of text on people's health records to identify reports of suicidality.[45] This, again, may be useful in predicting who may be most at risk of suicide. The real test of these new approaches will not necessarily be the accuracy of their predictions, but how well they can be combined with strategies to prevent suicide.

Like risk of self-harm, suicide risk can fluctuate daily and even hourly, depending on what is happening in the person's life. Temporal trends have been observed. Researchers studying social media found that suicide-related posts occur most frequently on Mondays, with an early-morning peak. This precedes the time of day when suicide attempts and deaths most commonly occur. Gaining greater insight into these weekly and daily rhythms could help us to inform public health campaigns and target support and interventions.[46]

RISK FACTORS

There has been considerable research into possible risk factors for suicide as a means to help support those who are vulnerable. No single factor is responsible for suicide and a number have been found to be influential, including genetic vulnerability and psychiatric, psychological, familial, social and cultural factors. These must all be considered in any preventative approach. The media, and more recently the internet, play important roles. Prevention needs to include universal measures, as well as those targeted specifically at high-risk groups.[47]

'Over the last 20 years we have come a long way in how we discuss suicide in the media, but there is more to do in terms of generating a real understanding. There are still a lot of myths around suicide and, although the number of people who believe those myths is getting smaller, each myth still persists and influences how we deal with suicide in society.'

PROFESSOR RORY O'CONNOR

Social context: lack of social cohesion and environmental factors

- Geographical location
- Sociocultural norms
- Disruption to social structure or values
- Economic turmoil
- Social isolation
- Media reporting
- Access to lethal means
- Poor access to mental health services

Distal factors

| Early-life adversity | Epigenic changes | Genetics | Family history |

Lasting alterations to gene expression

Developmental factors

Personality traits

| Genetic and epigenic factors | Chronic substance misuse | Impulsive aggression | Negative affect | Cognitive deficits |

Increased vulnerability to stress

Proximal factors

Life events → Psychopathology ← Biological, psychological, genetic and epigenic factors

Depressed and dysregulated mood, hopelessness and entrapment

Acute substance abuse

Behavioural disinhibition

| Thoughts about death | Acts of self-harm with intent to die | Death |

| Suicidal ideation (2.0-2.1%) | Suicidal attempt (0.3-0.4%) | Suicidal attempt (10.6 per 100,000 population) |

FACTORS THAT INFLUENCE SUICIDE

Using data from the Avon Longitudinal Study of Parents and Children, researchers studied young people who were thinking about suicide or engaging in non-suicidal self-harm to assess which factors may make them at risk of suicidal behaviour at the age of 21. The findings suggest that asking about substance use, self-harm, sleep and exposure to self-harm could inform risk assessments, and might help clinicians to identify adolescents who are at greatest risk of attempting suicide in the future.[48]

DIFFERENT AND ISOLATED

Rates of suicidal thoughts and attempts are higher among LGBT+ young people than their heterosexual peers. Through in-depth interviews, researchers have explored how young people with lived experience of suicidal distress make sense of the relationship between homophobia, biphobia and transphobia, and suicidal thoughts and attempts.[49] The findings show that suicide can be understood as a response to stigma, discrimination and harassment. These produce a sense of entrapment, rejection and isolation that can often form the basis of suicidal thoughts and action.

Research has also examined the prevalence of people with autism spectrum disorder, known to be vulnerable to mental health conditions, among those who have died by suicide. A study in England showed that autism and autistic traits are over-represented in those who die by suicide in England, accounting for 41.4 per cent of total suicide deaths.[50]

Support needs to be tailored to autistic people, especially given that many report being excluded from services and receiving inappropriate support and treatment for mental health problems. Wider societal issues, such as social exclusion and isolation, poverty, unemployment, trauma and abuse, are also significantly more common among autistic people than non-autistic people, and these issues further increase their risk of attempting suicide.

Loneliness is another area that has come to the fore in the study of suicide. Research shows that loneliness predicts both suicidal thinking and death by suicide, and that depression could be the factor that mediates the relationship.[51]

TRANSITION FROM SUICIDAL THOUGHTS AND ACTIONS

When thinking about risk, it's important to recognise that the factors influencing suicidal thoughts may be different to those influencing suicide attempts. To be able to provide better support, it's essential that we understand the distinctions between these phases and what influences someone to move from thoughts to actions.

Research shows that there are differences between men and women in terms of their pathways to suicide. Women, for example, report more suicidal ideation and suicide attempts than men. In both men and women a history of hospitalisation for mental illness is linked to suicide attempts, highlighting the need for monitoring of risk following discharge. The long-term impact of life experiences such as childhood adversity is also linked to suicide attempts in both sexes.[52]

MYTHS AROUND SUICIDE

Research is improving our understanding of the complex journey that brings people to suicide and how we might be able to change the nature and direction of that path. Despite this increase in awareness and understanding, there still exist a number of myths around the subject, and these can hinder progress towards suicide prevention.

Some of these myths are more harmful and rigid than others. One that is proving particularly hard to dispel is the belief that if you talk to, or ask, someone about suicide it may plant the idea of suicide in their head or encourage them to have suicidal thoughts or to act on them. There is no evidence behind this. There is, however, evidence that if you ask someone if they are suicidal it may start a conversation that could help them get the support they need, or even save their life.

'I don't dispute that it's difficult to ask about suicide and most people's biggest fear when they ask someone if they are suicidal is that they say "yes". If they do say yes it's crucial to be non-judgemental, not to minimise and to try to empathise. That sense of validation, containment and connection is so important. It's not your responsibility to solve their problems, but this is the start of a conversation that could be the chink of light for them. A sense of compassion and common humanity is key.'

PROFESSOR RORY O'CONNOR

Another common myth is that an improvement in emotional state equates to a lessened risk of suicide. Sadly, the reality is that people who have been depressed and suicidal often appear recovered in the days or weeks before they die. This lift in mood offers a false reassurance to others that the person is getting better, when in fact their mood has lifted because they have decided on suicide as a means to end their pain. With this lift in mood comes the capacity and motivation to plan and carry out the suicidal act.

'If somebody gets better because their crisis has resolved or their medication or psychological therapies are working, you can understand that. It's the unexpected increase or unexplained lift in mood that, when people have been suicidal, can be a concern. It stresses the importance of vigilance.'

PROFESSOR RORY O'CONNOR

MOTIVATIONAL AND VOLITIONAL PHASES

As suicide is a behaviour, we can gain an insight into what influences its passage using behavioural models. Researchers have developed a model that aims to better identify not only who will or won't develop suicidal thoughts, but who will act on these thoughts and when. This can inform clinical and preventative work.

The Integrated Motivational-Volitional (IVM) model draws on existing evidence on factors known to influence suicide. It proposes that suicidal behaviour results from a complex interplay of these factors and, from this, comes the intention for suicide (motivational phase). According to the model suicidal

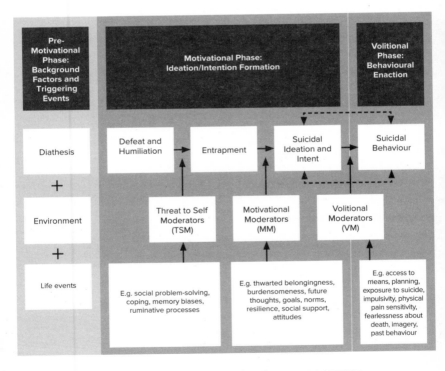

THE INTENTIONAL MOTIVATIONAL-VOLITIONAL (IVM) MODEL OF SUICIDE

thinking emerges from a sense of entrapment, caused by feelings of defeat and humiliation, which are further driven by feelings of loss, shame and rejection, often linked to stress.

Feelings of powerlessness and of not being able to escape from mental pain are key to suicidal behaviour. Researchers have developed an entrapment scale, used to identify these feelings, which can be used in research and clinical practice.[53] High levels of entrapment combined with high levels of loneliness have been found to increase someone's risk of suicide considerably.[54]

THE 4-TERM ENTRAPMENT SCALE (SHORT-FORM)

I often have the feeling that I would just like to run away

I feel powerless to change things

I feel trapped inside myself

I feel I'm in a deep hole that I can't get out of

'Clinicians and policymakers have told me that they find this model valuable but, more importantly, people with lived experience have said that the model is really helpful because it enables them to understand how they feel the way they do. And given that one of the dominating characteristics of the suicidal mind is ambivalence between living and dying, this enables a depiction of how the intensity of the suicidal thoughts comes and goes because – in the moment of desperation – the person thinks these thoughts will never end and the model can be used to help people and those around them make sense of this.'

PROFESSOR RORY O'CONNOR

The move from motivation to volition is key to understanding suicide attempts. The IVM model proposes that there are eight factors associated with crossing the precipice between thoughts and acts. These eight volitional factors help depict the transition and range from being able to access the means to die by suicide and impulsive behaviour, to mental imagery around death and knowing a friend or family member who has died by suicide (see the table on p.298).[55, 56]

'So if somebody is talking about suicide, you can look at these eight factors and try to formulate who's at risk, how can we work with them to keep an individual safe. Approaches like safety planning can be used at this stage because this helps a person identify their warning signs and coping responses, which might be keeping your environment safe and keeping the distance between you and that method as big as possible.'

PROFESSOR RORY O'CONNOR

HORMONAL STRESS RESPONSE AND SUICIDE

More recently, researchers have investigated the possible role of the hormone cortisol in suicidal thoughts and behaviour. Cortisol is released in response to stress, increasing sugars in the bloodstream, enhancing the brain's use of glucose and increasing the availability of substances that repair tissues. It also curbs functions such as digestion or reproduction that would be unnecessary or hindering in a fight-or-flight situation.

There is evidence that people who are suicidal do not release cortisol in the same way as people who are not suicidal. In lab studies, researchers found that people who had attempted suicide produced lower levels of cortisol in response to stress compared to those who thought about suicide and those who had neither thought about nor attempted suicide. The group with the lowest levels of cortisol were those people who had attempted suicide most recently and who had a family history of a suicide attempt.[57]

Out of the lab, researchers have also measured (using saliva tests) people's so-called 'cortisol awakening response' immediately after waking in the morning. These studies show that people with suicidal histories release less cortisol in the morning, as do people with psychological risk factors such as worry, perfectionism and impulsivity.[58] The next step will be to find out more about the mechanisms that link these different aspects of suicide risk.

Having this blunted cortisol response does not mean that someone becomes less stressed, but that they are less physiologically prepared to deal with stress when it comes along. Researchers suggest there is a 'wear and tear' process occurring. This idea is supported by findings that show that age influences cortisol response in people who are suicidal. For those under 40 there is a positive relationship between cortisol and suicide attempts, indicating that they are hyper-responsive in their hormonal reaction to stress. In people over the age of 40, meanwhile, this relationship changes and less cortisol is released. It appears that, for people in this group who are thinking about or attempting suicide, the body is overcome by stress and releases less cortisol. This dysregulation of the cortisol response creates a perfect storm of risk factors, whereby the hormonal response is coupled with unbearable mental pain and a sense of entrapment.

Given that research has also shown that people who have experienced trauma have a lower cortisol response, it adds to our understanding of the possible pathway to suicide.[59] It also highlights the importance of early intervention and protecting those children and young people who have experienced or are vulnerable to trauma. Trauma can be experienced repeatedly over a lifespan, which ties in with the idea of wear and tear reducing the cortisol response.

APPROACHES TO SUICIDE PREVENTION

Over the last 20 years, there has been a growing focus on ways to prevent suicide that have recognised its multifaceted nature and the diverse range of factors at play.

Evidence shows that cognitive behavioural therapy (CBT) can be effective in helping to change thinking patterns that may lead to suicidal behaviour, and models such as CBT-SP[60] have been developed specifically to this end. Dialectical behaviour therapy (DBT), which is based on CBT, has also been found to be effective. It is specially adapted for people who feel emotions very intensely, helping them to understand that two things that seem opposite can both be true. These approaches work at the motivational stage of the IVM model to reduce the sense of defeat, entrapment and humiliation.

The Attempted Suicide Short Intervention Program (ASSIP) is an innovative therapy that has been shown to be highly effective in reducing the risk of further attempts of suicide.[61, 62] The emphasis is on the therapeutic relationship, with four therapy sessions followed by continuing regular contact by letter.

Another approach that has had success is the Collaborative Assessment and Management of Suicidality (CAMS),[63] which focuses on the management of suicidal thoughts through the relationship with the clinician, who aims to understand the patient's suffering from an empathetic, non-judgemental perspective.

Common to these various psychosocial approaches to prevention is a safety planning component. Safety planning is a tool for helping people navigate suicidal feelings, and can be a way for the person and those supporting them to plan how to communicate and check in with each other. It may include a list of signs that indicate someone is in crisis, internal coping strategies, the names of friends and family who can help them navigate a crisis, lists of mental health professionals and agencies to call, and ways to make it harder for the person to harm themselves.

Aligned with the IMV model, researchers have developed a volitional help sheet, another brief intervention, which people can use when they have a suicidal trigger or warning sign. This helps them to respond with different behaviours or thoughts, as discussed with a healthcare professional. The help sheet supports them in identifying alternative behaviours. Again, this approach aims to challenge suicidal thoughts and interfere with the transition from thoughts to action as a means of keeping people safe in moments of acute crisis. Suicidality waxes and wanes and, if it is possible to get someone safely through a period of high-intent suicidal thoughts, they could enter a lower-risk period where more long-term work can be done.

Lifestyle is important in suicide prevention, because behaviours such as drinking and drug abuse can influence someone's transition from thoughts to action. People usually engage with these lifestyle choices as a means of dealing with mental pain and distress, but they actually reduce the person's cognitive ability to solve the problems at the source of their suffering. They also compound many other mental health conditions and impact negatively on quality of life. Community mental health programmes around social skills training can help incorporate education on lifestyle and ultimately reduce suicide risk.[64]

Thanks to research, our understanding of all aspects of suicide is improving: its prevalence, the factors that influence suicidal thoughts and behaviour, and what influences the move from thoughts to action. We are also gaining greater insight into what might be happening at a hormonal level, which may help us to predict vulnerability and fluctuation in risk. Ultimately, this knowledge will inform prevention and support.

As with other areas of mental health research, the focus needs to be on the underlying mechanisms and how they contribute to risk. This can help in the development of more personalised approaches for people of different sexes, sexualities, neurodiversities and ethnic backgrounds. Central to this is seeking the input and involvement of people with lived experience at every step of the process.

MYTHS SURROUNDING SUICIDE

Those who talk about suicide are not at risk

All suicidal people are mentally ill or depressed

Suicide occurs without warning

Asking about suicide plants the idea in someone's head

Suicidal people clearly want to die

When someone becomes suicidal they will always remain suicidal

Suicide is inherited

Suicidal behaviour is motivated by attention seeking

Suicide is caused by a single factor

Suicide cannot be prevented

Only people of a particular social class die by suicide

Improvement in emotional state means lessened risk of suicide

Thinking about suicide is rare

People who attempt suicide by a low-lethality method are not serious about killing themselves

Suicidal ideation and intent

Access to means
Does individual have ready access to likely means of suicide?

Planning (if-then plans)
Has individual formulated a plan for suicide?

Exposure to suicide or suicidal behaviour
Has a family member/friend engaged in suicidal behaviour?

Impulsivity
Does individual tend to act impulsively/on spur of moment?

Physical pain/sensitivity/endurance
Has the individual high (increased) physical pain endurance?

Fearlessness about death
Is individual fearful about death/has this changed?

Mental imagery
Does individual describe visualising dying/after death?

Past suicidal behaviour
Has the individual a history of suicide attempts or self-harm?

Suicidal behaviour

FACTORS THAT MOVE PEOPLE FROM SUICIDE IDEATION AND INTENT TO
SUICIDE BEHAVIOUR

'We need to develop treatments and approaches that consider underlying mechanisms, tailored and informed by those who truly understand suicidal thoughts and behaviours; namely those who have been suicidal and those who have been bereaved. Also, there is a need to look at new models of service delivery that go where people are, rather than expecting those people to come to us.'

PROFESSOR RORY O'CONNOR

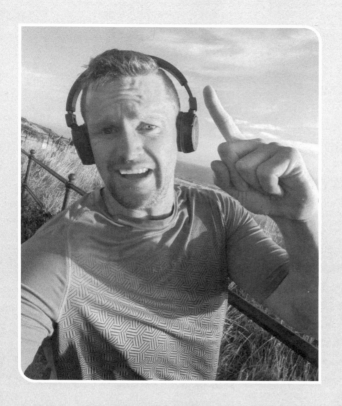

Peter 'Taf' Mather is the owner of Sky-High Drop Zone in Durham and the founder of the charity Uplift, which supports skydivers struggling with their mental health. He has represented Great Britain in formation skydiving at world level and has won multiple national medals.

I've struggled with substance abuse since the age of 18. I've been addicted to drugs and had a heart attack at the age of 21 because of a cocaine overdose. I worked as a bartender and I fell into the trap of partying, drinking and taking drugs. I realise now that really I was running away from a feeling that I was never good enough. I couldn't get past it. Even when I'm very good at things it was never enough.

HIDING FROM THE PAIN

When I took up skydiving it was a way to try to transform my life. It is an amazing sport, but it involves chasing adrenaline and unfortunately it brings with it a lot of alcohol and other substances. And I just fell into this trap again. For me I don't think it matters whether it was skydiving or something else – the way I see it the same thing would have happened because I just couldn't admit I had a major problem with self-doubt and I was always trying to please people. Just like the drugs and the drink, I used skydiving as pain relief and I was always trying to get away from the mental pain.

I've had an amazing life, but I've done some horrendous things and met some horrendous people. I've ruined relationships with my family and people around me. It all boils down to self-esteem. I'd be using cocaine and drinking and would be surrounded by girls, thinking, 'this is the life I should want to live'. Yet all it did was make me unhappy.

SUICIDE

There were many times when I thought about suicide but never did it. I thought about it quite a lot when I was skydiving. I wondered whether I could just smack my canopy into the ground or hit a building. What would happen? What would people do? In 2020, I started a skydiving business, and three days later the

pandemic hit, sending me £2.7 million into debt overnight.
I started using cocaine every day of the week; I just didn't
care any more.

When the relationship with my girlfriend ended, I got to the
point where I was prepared to die. I just didn't know what else
to do. I stood on a cliff edge and thought, 'what have I got to
live for?' Something in my head told me not to jump, but to
drive the car off the cliff instead, so I got in the car and
visualised doing it. Then the phone rang. It was my business
partner. He didn't even know what was going on but all he
needed to say was, 'Are you all right big man?' and then I just
broke down and started crying.

At the time he didn't even know that he saved my life but when
he asked me that simple question I just felt this massive
empathy. And when I cried it broke the pattern of always trying
to be all right and to please people. It completely broke the
pattern.

PUTTING CHANGES IN PLACE

That was the start of the changes in my life. The first thing I did
was ask for help and admitting I wasn't all right was the biggest
step. I saw a counsellor and hired a lifestyle coach. I stopped
drinking and taking drugs and I've been clean now for two
years.

You find your own path to change but I do think that what most
people need is that empathy with themselves and a belief that
they can change. And when that happens you don't need the
alcohol or the drugs or suicide to take you away from reality and
from dealing with your problems. The first step for me was
overcoming the pain of admitting I have a problem, and to do
that I needed empathy and the right environment with the right
people around me.

I'm a great believer in the value of habits and rituals and routines, so I started to change my bad habits around drugs and lifestyle and found ways to be grateful each day, to thank myself and feel an important part of this world. For me it's also about outwardly committing to change. In some ways I think I'm selfish because the more I talk about how I have changed my life, the more I cannot go back to the way I was. I'm putting myself out there and saying I'm this guy that's changed my life. And I do that because I must never go back. So I tell my story and I've created this charity around mental health and skydiving because that keeps me going forward and reminds me of the reasons why I do it.

I'm determined to stop people dying by suicide in our sport because we've had a lot in the last two years. We have also had people who self-harm and who use substances. So my goal for the charity is based on developing a support network that people can go to and talk and be understood.

FUTURE DEVELOPMENTS

Self-destructive behaviour is complex, difficult to comprehend from the outside, and it affects not only the individual but those around them. Because of a lack of knowledge and understanding of these issues in society, many people fear even talking about them, which allows myths to be perpetuated.

Through research, we are gaining greater insight into the triggers and mechanisms involved in self-destructive behaviours and how we can better help people who use them in order to cope. The more we understand, however, the clearer it becomes that every experience of these behaviours is different and valid. They demonstrate the intricacy and interdependency of factors that influence mental health conditions in general. Self-destructive behaviours also highlight the negative impacts of stigma, misunderstanding and fear on a person's ability to seek and receive help, causing isolation and closing down the conversations that could ultimately save their life.

When someone close to us uses self-destructive behaviour, especially when that leads to devastating consequences, it is natural to want to know the cause. Having something clear-cut to blame is in itself a way of coping. The reality, however, is not so simple. Research can help to shed light on why certain people engage in self-destructive behaviours, but it can't provide all the answers.

INTERDEPENDENCY OF BEHAVIOURS

Although in this chapter we have described three forms of self-destructive behaviour separately, research has shown that they are very much interlinked. Rather than describing people in terms of the behaviour they are engaging in, it may be more useful to consider their journey and what leads them to different behaviours at different times. Self-destructive behaviours are fluid over time, making them challenging to define and study. However, it is not impossible.

For some people, self-harm takes on the nature of an addictive behaviour. Indeed, research looking at social media forums has shown that people who self-harm describe their experience as an 'addiction', citing cravings or urges to self-harm, as well as escalating severity,[65] reflecting a form of tolerance. When talking about their self-harm, people also frequently use language and concepts common to addiction recovery, such as 'getting clean', 'relapse' and 'recovery'.

Self-harm and addiction have also been cited as risk factors for suicide. Young people who use substances or alcohol and who have a mental health condition are at greatest risk of suicide, especially if they are male.[66] In 2019, one in five problem gamblers thought about suicide and one in twenty made a suicide attempt.[67]

Although most adolescents who think about suicide or engage in non-suicidal self-harm will not act on it, it is still an indicator that suicide will occur later in life.[68]

Understanding this interdependency of behaviours and the fluidity in risk can help us to avoid pigeonholing people into certain types of behaviour. We can work with them according to the factors influential at the time to understand why their self-destructive behaviour seems the best option for coping and look to develop healthier alternatives.

One of the major challenges in identifying, comprehending and treating self-destructive behaviours is how hidden they remain, by individuals and by society. From a policy viewpoint this makes it difficult to understand the scale, trends and location of the problem, which in turn can mean people don't get the support or resources they require.

BIG DATA AND NATURAL LANGUAGE PROCESSING

The use of large electronic datasets from healthcare, educational and social services is enabling researchers to better identify how much and where self-destructive behaviour is happening. This is often data that is collected routinely, rather than offered volitionally through studies that recruit people engaging in self-destructive behaviours.

By mining and linking these datasets, researchers are starting to connect the dots and identify common traits and factors between people who self-harm, are addicted to substances and activities, and who think about, or die by suicide.

Innovative ways of connecting and analysing across datasets is helping us to map out what influences self-destructive behaviour and how we can help people at the right place, at the right time. For example, a wealth of data exists in people's health records, and NLP approaches are allowing researchers to tap into these rich seams of information.

Algorithms are being developed to harness more value from NLP,[69] potentially enabling us to identify those people most vulnerable to suicide. NLP has also been developed to identify self-harm in women who are pregnant or who have recently had a baby.[70] This is a very vulnerable group and one where self-destructive behaviours are likely to be hidden for fear of judgement and repercussions for themselves and their children. These data analysis approaches can also take a longitudinal view over time, capturing fluctuations of behaviours, which can help to inform timely support services.

In the world of gambling, academic partnerships with the online gambling industry are enabling real-time tracking of gamblers' behaviour, providing a rich dataset on how people gamble. This tracking is currently limited to just one site, so can't provide an overarching view of individuals' behaviour, but it is still potentially very valuable insight.[71]

SOCIAL MEDIA

Recent media coverage, involving young people who have self-harmed or committed suicide after viewing content on social media, has highlighted the role of these platforms in self-destructive behaviours. New research is investigating this in more depth, working with young people and tracking their social media interactions, self-harm and mental health over time. The hope is that this will provide greater clarity on the positive and negative impacts of social media on young people and help to shape future policy in this area.

Social media can be a rich source of data, as researchers can track when and where people share posts on self-destructive behaviour. There are, for example, certain forums such as SuicideWatch (a moderated online community on Reddit) aimed specifically at individuals who are either at risk of suicide, or who know someone who is. Analysis of posts on this forum shows a clear variation in behaviour throughout the week and during the day.[72] It was research on posts from self-harm forums on Reddit that demonstrated the addictive-type language that is used in these communities,[73] providing insight into the driving forces behind self-harm.

FOCUS ON MECHANISMS

Researchers are striving to better understand the different mechanisms (biological, cognitive and social) that underlie self-destructive behaviours. As with other areas of mental health, these are unlikely to switch on and off in the lead-up to, and after, the behaviour. Instead they influence behaviour incrementally and overlay with others.

Studies examining changes in brain chemicals, hormones and genetics (through epigenetics) are beginning to reveal some important insights into these behaviours. More research is needed to understand them better and, perhaps more importantly, to explore whether they are shared with different forms of behaviour. These studies do not suggest a singular biological approach to treatment or support, but they are providing an improved understanding of these conditions and helping to fill in some of the gaps in the big picture.

Describing the details of the thought processes and biases behind these behaviours is important in understanding why they develop in the first place. These thinking patterns are laid down over time, so if we can understand how and why this happens we may be able to introduce healthier alternatives before the harmful patterns become embedded.

Social processes are also important to investigate. Research into the influence of accessibility on addiction, for example, is helping to influence programmes and actions to limit access to harmful substances and activities. There is a difficult line to tread in order to raise awareness of self-destructive behaviours without normalising them.

TECHNOLOGICAL INNOVATIONS

Technological advances are enabling innovative approaches to help people manage addictions, self-harm and suicidal behaviours. One example is the use of virtual reality to enable addicts to enter, virtually, into a situation where they might come across the substance or activity they're addicted to. There, they can begin to unpick the related thoughts and actions with a therapist. A similar approach, using images and videos, has been used previously in CBT, but with virtual reality the situations feel much more real, so cravings and urges are more likely to be triggered. Research has shown that VR gaming induces a gambling urge comparable to the one people experience playing with real money, and therapists can identify about twice as many problematic thoughts.[74]

Researchers have also proposed that virtual reality has a potential application in the identification and possible treatment of non-suicidal self-harm. With its immersive visuals, it may induce the emotions known to trigger self-harm, enabling individuals to talk through their thoughts in a safe and supported environment.

Technology has also enabled new opportunities for harm reduction, including the development of the antidote naloxone (see the section on addiction, p.277). Researchers are also investigating the potential use of remote sensors to detect overdoses, enabling quick action to be taken. During an overdose, one of the most serious indications is respiratory depression (slow and shallow breathing), and this could possibly be detected and monitored.

Ultimately, many of these new approaches are about giving people more choice, independence and respect in managing their own behaviour, rather than suggesting that the only possible option is to cease it altogether. For such approaches to be successful they will need to go hand in hand with a shift in public attitude, so that any empowerment feels genuine and can lead to positive and long-term changes in behaviour.

WHERE NOW?

IN AN EMERGENCY, OR A SITUATION WHERE THERE IS IMMEDIATE THREAT TO LIFE, YOU SHOULD ALWAYS DIAL 999.

If you have been struggling with thoughts of self-destruction, addiction, suicide, or you have been deliberately hurting yourself, there is help available.

In the first instance, contacting your GP is always the best route to getting help and support. You can also reach out to the NHS 111 service if you can't get through to your GP.

If you are not ready to speak to your GP, or if you cannot wait for an appointment and need to speak to someone urgently, then you should call the Samaritans. Their number, along with other relevant sources of support, is listed below.

Talking to your GP about self-harm and suicide

If you are worried about speaking to your GP on your own about wanting to hurt yourself then it is possible to ask a trusted friend or loved one to go with you for support.

Your GP will listen to you and may ask you some questions about how you are feeling. If you have been self-harming, they may want to look at your injuries.

They will then discuss with you the best course of action for you. This might include talking therapies, group support therapies, or medication. They may also refer you to a local community mental health team for further assessment.

In addition to referring you to a specialist, your GP might discuss making a 'safety plan' with you. This is a plan for when those feelings of self-destruction are strongest and is designed to help keep you safe. This might involve having a trusted contact you can call when you are feeling low, or ensuring that you don't have immediate access to ways to hurt yourself.

If you are worried about someone else:

If you think that someone is in immediate danger you should call 999. If someone tells you they are having thoughts of self-harm or suicide then it is vital you believe them. Suicidal thoughts cannot be seen from the outside and just because someone doesn't present as being depressed, stressed or suicidal doesn't mean that they are not at risk. Thoughts of suicide and self-harm can come in waves and, while someone might appear to be fine in one moment, they might start having intrusive thoughts of hurting themselves in the next moment.

You should listen to that person and ask questions if necessary. Try not to offer opinions or share your own experiences, as for some people that can be interpreted as minimising their feelings.

You should, however, encourage them to speak to their GP. You could also offer to accompany them as it can be very scary to speak to a doctor alone about thoughts of self-harm.

If you are worried that someone is suicidal or that they are self-harming, then it is OK to ask them directly. You will not make someone suicidal by asking them if they have ever considered harming themselves.

If you are having problems with addiction

There are many types of addiction, both physical and psychological. For example, while some people may become addicted to substances, others may become addicted to shoplifting or, as discussed in this chapter, gambling. The most important thing to remember is that addiction is a treatable condition and there is help available.

If you feel that you are drinking too much, using drugs too often, or if you have a behaviour that you just cannot seem to stop, then you could reach out to one of the organisations listed below, who can give you specialist advice.

You can also search the NHS website for a list of local resources; just search for 'addiction support' on NHS.uk.

Alternatively, you can speak to your GP, who will be able to recommend a local service or organisation for you to contact. This might include support groups such as Narcotics or Alcoholics Anonymous, attending therapy sessions or even in some extreme cases attending a rehabilitation clinic.

Here are some other sources of advice and support:

Samaritans.org

The Samaritans can be reached 24/7, 365 days a year by dialling 116 123. Not much of a talker? You can also email them any time at jo@samaritans.org and someone will get back to you within 24 hours.

Nightline.ac.uk

For higher education students Nightline offer volunteer-run telephone support. Each university or educational establishment's telephone number is different, so please visit their website for more information.

Themix.org.uk

For under 25s, the Mix offers support on a variety of issues including self-harm and addiction. They can be reached between 4pm and 11pm every day on 0808 808 4994.

Nshn.co.uk

The National Self Harm Network is an online support forum that provides information, resources and immediate distraction for individuals who self-harm and their friends and family.

ForwardTrust.org.uk

As well as online resources and information about how to move forward from addiction issues, the Forward Trust offer a web-based chat service, Monday to Friday from 9am to 3pm, for anyone struggling with addiction.

TalkToFrank.com

FRANK offer advice about drugs and substance abuse issues. They offer a helpline that anyone can call, including if you are worried about someone else's drug use. 0300 123 6600.

HumanKindCharity.org.uk

Humankind tailor their services and support depending on an individual's complex health and social needs. You can email them at info@humankindcharity.org.uk or call them on 01325 731 160.

the experts

RORY O'CONNOR

Rory O'Connor is director of the Suicidal Behaviour Research Laboratory at the University of Glasgow, one of the leading suicide and self-harm research groups internationally. He is also president of the International Association for Suicide Prevention. A registered health psychologist, he is also involved in policy work. From a young age he was always fascinated by mental health, and he remembers hearing people talk about depression but not understanding why some people were affected and others weren't. This interest continued and he went on to study psychology at university, writing a dissertation that focused on depression. Through this experience he discovered his love of the research process and, after finishing his undergraduate degree, he started a PhD in suicide, drawing on his previous work on depression and hopelessness. Sadly, the person who brought him into the field took his own life, and a close friend also died by suicide in 2008. This further highlighted to him the challenges in prevention and the urgency of researching suicide to address these challenges. He has continued to research suicide for the last 25 years and is the recipient of the 2023 American Foundation for Suicide Prevention research award.

MARK GRIFFITHS

Mark Griffiths is Distinguished Professor in the School of Social Sciences at Nottingham Trent University. He is a chartered psychologist and director of the International Gaming Research Unit. He mostly teaches on areas related to his research interests, on various undergraduate and postgraduate psychology programmes. His main teaching interests are in the areas of abnormal, social and health psychology with particular emphasis on behavioural addictions (gambling addiction, videogame addiction, internet addiction, sex addiction, exercise addiction, work addiction, etc.), cyberpsychology and the psychology of sexual behaviour. In 2006, he was awarded the British Psychological Society's highest teaching honour, the Excellence in Teaching of Psychology Award. In addition to his teaching and research, Professor Griffiths is also a gaming consultant and works with the gaming industry to promote responsible gambling, social responsibility, harm minimisation, and player protection. He is also a freelance journalist and writes for many national and international newspapers and magazines.

ANN JOHN

Ann John is a professor in public health and psychiatry at the Swansea University Medical School and co-director of DATAMIND, the HDR-UK hub for mental health data. Ann leads a research programme with a focus on mental health data science Including the MQ-funded Adolescent Mental Health Data Platform. It was when she started reading medicine that she developed an interest in studying health at a population level and epidemiology. She came top of her year in the sociology exam and was offered a place to do an integrated BSc in sociology. This experience changed the way she looked at medicine, in terms of placing it in the broader context of society and culture. After she finished medical school she worked in A&E and then went into general practice, where she developed a strong interest in mental health. She kept this focus when she moved into public health and then research, studying anxiety, depression and self-harm, which are conditions often seen in primary care. Throughout her career she has always been passionate about translating research into policy and practice in order to improve people's lives, particularly in the prevention of self-harm and suicide. She has advised on storylines for a number of TV productions including *Coronation Street* and *This is Going to Hurt.* She is a trustee of the Samaritans.

SPOTLIGHT ON AGEING HAPPILY

Getting older is a transition – albeit a gradual one – that can bring with it feelings of loss and sadness. It can trigger questions around our identity if we no longer feel that we are the same person and capable of the same activities. With this can come reflections on what we have in life, which can impact self-esteem and mood.

Ageing encompasses both physical and mental health. Advances in medicine and healthcare have led to increased life expectancies, but ageing is still accompanied by frailty and shifts in how we think and feel. Researchers are investigating the factors that influence age-related changes in our mood and our thinking to try to unlock how we can age healthily and happily.

Like many aspects of our health, ageing is a very individual process, depending on factors ranging from the biological to the social. We are learning more about the physiological and hormonal processes involved in ageing, but how we age also depends on our perceptions of growing older. Modern society tends to focus on youth and suggestions on how to keep young.

To understand how our brain ages and possible ways to enable a better ageing process, researchers are working with large datasets that follow people over time from middle to old age to identify those factors that influence how we age. They are also investigating what happens in the brain at a cellular level and the different aspects of our lifestyle and environment that affect this, such as diet, exercise, sleep and stress.

GROWING NEW BRAIN CELLS

As we develop from foetuses into babies, through childhood and into young adults we are continually growing new brain cells or neurones. This is not a surprise. However, what is not so well known is that adults can also grow new brain cells – through a process known as adult neurogenesis.

This was initially discovered by researchers in the 1960s[1] when they showed that adult rats could produce new neurones. At the time there was not much recognition of this discovery, but in the 1990s new tools that could trace how stem cells develop into specialised brain or muscle cells allowed researchers to demonstrate the process of neurogenesis in the human brain; more specifically, in a brain area called the hippocampus, which plays an important role in memory, emotion and mood.

Since then researchers have shown that adults generate about 700 new neurones per day in the hippocampus.[2] This may seem quite a small number in comparison to the billions of neurones that exist in the brain, but these new neurones that are created in adults are quite specific to the hippocampus, where new brain cells can have a large impact due to the connections they make.

By the time we turn 50 it is estimated we will have exchanged all the hippocampus neurones we were born with with neurones that have been created during adulthood.

Due to the hippocampus's role in memory, mood and emotion, these findings suggest that through a better understanding of the mechanisms that influence adult neurogenesis we could help improve or maintain our memory and mood as we age.

LINKING NEUROGENESIS TO THINKING PROCESSES AND MOOD

Researchers have found ways to block or stop the process of neurogenesis in adult animals, which enables us to study its role in ageing. This type of research has shown that less neurogenesis results in a decline in learning. More recently, researchers have also shown that limiting neurogenesis also prevents animals from completing tasks of pattern separation.[3] Skills in performing these types of task are involved in distinguishing memories that are similar to each other and linked to our ability to remember where we put everyday objects such as keys, wallets and phones from a selection of familiar locations. Researchers have suggested that difficulties in differentiating memories of similar patterns could lead to the automatic negative thinking patterns that are part of depression.[4]

The process of creating new neurones as adults naturally slows down with age and alongside this comes impaired learning and memory abilities.[5,6] Moreover, production of new neurones as adults is reduced by stressful experiences, particularly when this stress is long-term and constant, which is linked to depression. Confirming this link to depression, studies have also shown that many antidepressant treatments enhance and are dependent on neurogenesis.[7]

DIET, EXERCISE, SLEEP AND NEUROGENESIS

There is a growing body of evidence demonstrating a relationship between lifestyle factors, such as exercise and diet,[8] and how our thought processes and mood change as we age.

Researchers have investigated the effect of exercise on adult neurogenesis in mice and shown that older mice who exercised on a wheel performed better on memory tasks and showed a slowing down in their natural reduction in the production of new neurones.[9]

Sleep influences the production of new neurones in adults. Restriction or disruption of sleep for long periods of time leads to a decrease in neurogenesis in mice.[10]

Diet is another important environmental factor and researchers have studied four different ways by which diet can have an impact: calorie intake, meal frequency, meal texture and meal content. Both reducing calories and extending the time between meals seems to encourage the birth of new neurones in rodents.[11,12] Interestingly, food texture also has an impact; animals fed with a soft diet, as opposed to a solid and hard diet, create fewer new neurones in the hippocampus.[13]

Changing what we eat and the content of our meals offers perhaps the most flexibility to influence the production of new neurones as adults. Some of the dietary factors identified in animals have been reflected in research with humans that has shown that certain dietary changes can impact learning and memory. This has been demonstrated by studying the natural variation in diets across populations[14] and connecting this with differences in thinking and mood as we grow older. In another approach research has given groups of people different diets and different regimes, showing that Mediterranean-type diets consisting largely of healthy oils, nuts, fruit and vegetables can improve our thinking processes.[15]

Researchers have studied a variety of bioactives and nutrients and shown they have increased the production of new neurones. This has been supported by research with humans that has shown improvements in thinking when diets are enhanced with flavonoids, which are found in foods such as cocoa and blueberries, curcumin, which is in the spice turmeric,[16] and omega 3 fatty acids, which are found in oily fish and nuts.

Research is also trying to pinpoint the genetic mechanisms that can explain the association between lifestyle and ageing in humans. Studies have identified so-called nutrient-sensing pathways in which particular genes provide a potential explanation for how diet influences the ageing of neural cells and our memory ability.

Findings from laboratory experiments can narrow down the possible genetic mechanisms, which can then be investigated in large datasets at a population level.[17] This has shown that variations in certain genes are associated with memory and that they are also instrumental in the relationship between memory, diet and exercise. The findings suggest that changes in lifestyle may be able to delay a decline in memory but that the effectiveness of these approaches will depend on an individual's genetic make-up. For example, adherence to a Mediterranean diet may be most beneficial for people with a specific genetic mutation, while increased exercise may be a better approach for participants with another type of variation.

AGEING, MOOD AND LIFESTYLE

Depression has been linked to growing older. As we age we experience more loss and grief, and we are potentially more likely to develop long-term health conditions. These could all be factors that influence our mood as we grow older and could be linked to changes in our brains.

Researchers have studied what happens to neurones in later-life depression and found that as depression develops there is not only a change in the processes involved in the creation of new neurones but those neurones that do develop are different in terms of shape and arrangement.[18] The researchers found evidence that dietary factors may be driving these changes.

There are several studies showing that those who have been diagnosed with depression engage in less physical activity[19] and that physical activity can successfully treat and prevent depressive symptoms.

However, the mechanisms behind these antidepressant effects are yet to be established. By collating existing evidence in this area, researchers have summarised possible key biological and psychosocial mechanisms through which physical activity exerts antidepressant effects.[20] This has shown that for more biological processes, exercise stimulates several processes that allow neurones to alter their structure and function, and this has been implicated in depression. Exercise also reduces inflammation and increases resilience to stress at a biological level.

On the psychosocial side, exercise promotes self-esteem and social support. A better understanding of how exercise takes effect can inform the way we design and put in place exercise-based approaches to managing depression. Researchers have mapped out a conceptual framework of the key biological and psychosocial mechanisms underlying the relationship between

Biological mechanisms

Neuroplasticity
- Molecular level neurotrophin release e.g. BDNF
- Cellular level changes in neurogenesis, angiogenisis, synaptogenesis, etc.
- Structural level changes in hippocampus, cortical regions and white matter
- Improved brain-wide vasculature

Neuroendocrine response
- Greater HPA regulation
- Changes in cortisol activity

Inflamation
- Decrease in basal pro-inflammatory markers, e.g. IL-6
- Increase in anti-inflammatory markers, e.g. IL-10
- Reduction in inflammation due to adipose tissue
- Changes in monocyte numbers and morphology

Oxidative stress
- Increased resilience to stress from excessive oxidative and nitrosative species

Psychosocial mechanisms

Self-esteem
- Improving physical self perceptions
- Positive body image perception

Social support
- More interaction and emotional disclosure
- Exposure to new social networks

Self-efficacy
- Skill mastery
- Transferable sense of coping with challenges
- Barrier self-efficacy

Physical activity

Depressive symptoms

Examples of moderators
- Age
- Biological profile e.g. IL-6 or BDNF levels
- Symptomology
- Length/severity of depression
- Psychosocial factors, e.g. body image or barriers to exercise
- Fitness level/charge
- Exercise protocol, e.g. intensity or duration of session
- Context of exercise, e.g. individual gym sessions or team sports
- Adherence to exercise

Examples of confounders
- Medication use
- Social deprivation
- Genetic factors, e.g. polygenic risk of depression
- Physical health status
- Stress
- Education
- Ethnicity
- Other psychiatric conditions
- Other health behaviours, e.g. sleep
- Trauma

MECHANISMS BEHIND EFFECTS OF PHYSICAL ACTIVITY ON DEPRESSION

physical activity and depressive symptoms, and the other factors that may influence it (see the figure opposite).

By summarising the findings from various studies investigating physical activity and anxiety, we can see that exercise does protect against anxiety, regardless of demographic variables and particularly for agoraphobia and post-traumatic disorders.[21]

GUT MICROBIOME, AGEING AND MENTAL HEALTH

With an estimated 1,018 microorganisms, the gut microbiome is responsible for multiple functions in bowel movement, digestion of food and absorption of nutrients. This not only has implications for our physical health but, because the brain and the gut work in a two-way manner, the microbiome could also impact stress, anxiety, depression and our thinking processes.[22]

Everyone's gut microbiota is different and depends on our genetics, stage of development and location.[23] The microbiome influences our immune and metabolic systems and could also be instrumental as a bridging mechanism in how environmental and lifestyle factors influence healthy ageing. However, the microbiome has a reciprocal relationship with age: it changes as we age and is altered by those diseases related to old age, but it can also modify negative changes that happen as a result of age.

Evidence is accumulating that gut microbiota may influence brain activity and behaviour, and a summary of research has shown a link between the microbes in the gastrointestinal tract and how individuals think. This suggests the gut–brain axis could be an important pathway in the understanding of mental health.[24] Several animal studies suggest that gut microbiota might have an impact on depression and research has shown that consumption of probiotics positively affects mood and anxiety in humans.[25] More recently researchers have identified 13 different types of microbe that may play a key role in depression.[26]

Although promising, gut microbiome studies have a long way to go. More laboratory experiments need to be done to find out how the composition, qualities or concentrations of gut microorganisms influence certain behaviours within the spectrum of mental health and illness. We are still far from establishing the role of these fantastic gut microbes in how we think but the hope is that, once we understand the specifics fully, they may provide a route to managing our mental health.

There is a lot of existing evidence that our lifestyle choices can affect our mental health as we age and provide a pathway to improvement, prevention and even treatment for those people who have been diagnosed with mental health disorders. This has been reflected in health policy, with NICE recommending physical activity as a way to treat depression and public health campaigns encouraging us to eat better and exercise more.

To many of us these recommendations around lifestyle for healthy ageing make intuitive sense, but research in this area is essential to ensure a greater understanding of the mechanisms, from the cellular to the social, on the ageing process. This in turn can inform current approaches that include lifestyle factors and provide more specific insight into future treatments for some of the negative aspects of ageing. As with all aspects of our mental health, approaches to healthy, happy ageing will need to work at different levels, encompassing the biological, cognitive and social aspects of growing older while placing the individual in the centre.

'After turning 70 there is this absolute, inescapable realisation that it's downhill from here and you are on the home stretch. The upside of this is that it makes me appreciate every single day much more intensely than I used to: there are things I used to take for granted that I now see as gifts. Gardening is really important to me but I dread the day when I can't manage our garden any more. At the back of my mind there is this fear of what's around the corner but it's more a fatalism than an anxiety. I don't want to do anything that would accelerate the process and spend any of this good time feeling unwell. I want to make the most of every day I've got.'

BILL BRYSON

'We do not have to age as our previous generations have aged, and to do this we have to radically update our thinking about wellness. We need to think about health holistically and become more interested in our biology and the ways in which exercise, diet and music affect our biology because we have a lot more control than we think over our health and wellness. By striving to learn more about how our biology affects our mental health we can become more empowered to manage it.'

DR JULIA JONES

CONNECTIONS BETWEEN LIFESTYLE AND AGEING IN THE HUMAN BRAIN

As it is not possible to directly study the process of neurogenesis in the human brain, researchers are applying their knowledge from animal studies and developing innovative approaches to unpick what is behind the effect of lifestyle factors on ageing processes in the human brain. For example, one study used blood samples from people over 65 to treat human stem cells taken from the hippocampus[27] in the laboratory. Stem cells are the cells that are yet to specialise into functions such as brain or muscular cells.

The researchers recorded the effects of the blood on production of neurones from these stem cells and then analysed data on these people over the next 10 to 15 years to link any impacts on neurogenesis with any decline in thought processes and possible onset of Alzheimer's. Using this method, researchers showed that the blood of those who went on to experience a decline in thought processes and/or a diagnosis of Alzheimer's resulted in the death of hippocampal stem cells, indicating that levels of neurogenesis can potentially predict the onset of cognitive problems with thinking 12 years prior to a diagnosis.

The study also showed that physical activity and nutrition were key factors that determined the severity of decline in thinking, where reduced physical activity and increased lack of nutrition both increased cell death, which in turn increased the risk for future decline in thinking skills.

OTHER SOURCES OF SUPPORT

Throughout this book we have listed many organisations that offer tailored support for a range of mental health issues.

Here are some more sources of advice and support that have either been founded, or just recommended by, some of the people featured in this book.

SportingForce.org

Sporting Force is run by Tommy Lowther, whose story features in Chapter 1. They run weekly support groups as well as ongoing support for ex-service personnel who are transitioning back into civilian life.

Myblackdog.co

My Black Dog run an online peer-to-peer chat service with volunteers who have all experienced depression themselves.

Acacia.org.uk

Acacia Family Support offer pre- and postnatal depression support services to parents. Rebecca Wooldridge, whose story featured in Chapter 4, found they were helpful to her.

UpliftSkydiving.com

Uplift was co-founded by Peter 'Taf' Mather, whose story features in Chapter 5. They offer support tailored to British skydivers and members of the British Parachute Association.

Participate.mqmentalhealth.org

You could also take part in research. Researchers regularly trial new interventions both in person and online through interviews and questionnaires.

By volunteering to take part, you could be a part of the next big breakthrough in mental health research.

Find out more about volunteering for research here: participate.mqmentalhealth.org

If you are experiencing difficulty with your mental health, MQ have compiled a list of varied resources where you can access immediate help on a range of different topics:

conclusion

BY PROFESSOR PETER B. JONES, DEPARTMENT OF PSYCHIATRY, UNIVERSITY OF CAMBRIDGE

It has been a pleasure and a privilege to be involved in the production of this book. It deals with a key human challenge: understanding how we create our conscious world through our brains and bodies, and what happens when this everyday miracle goes awry. We have a number of terms to describe this, including mental health problems, mental illness, mental disorders or a combination of them all. Regardless of the term we use, such problems are common and cause huge disability and burden for individuals, families, carers and for society. The statistics are eye-watering, not least because mental illnesses often emerge during childhood, adolescence or young adulthood. And we can all be affected in one way or another.

So why a pleasure and a privilege? The privilege comes from the candid, first-person accounts from people with lived experience of mental illness. Their experiences hold to account clinicians, other supporters and researchers, as well as providing the motivation for them to continue. I have often wondered about how best to join the voices of those with lived experience of mental illness and the professional experience of researchers in a conversation. As a reader of this book it is now you who can make the links, another rather special privilege I encountered when I read the chapters.

The pleasure has come through the passionate and clear accounts from all contributors: experts by experience and by profession (and note that there's quite an unspoken overlap). In these pages world-leading scientists have described their research into mental illness with optimism and commitment and experts by experience have provided their insight into what has helped and supported them. Many branches of human endeavour help us make sense of mental illness and it's fair to say that the overlaps and interdisciplinary touch-points are particularly informative. It is from these that new understanding, prevention strategies and therapies will arise from accumulating knowledge and novel insights. My own position is that psychology, neuroscience and medicine are key research pillars at the moment and I hope that one overarching message from the book is the value and promise of supporting the kind of high-quality mental health science you've read.

The book is bold and creative. New intersections within the mental health sciences are telling us how genes and environments interact, and how we can understand risk, resilience and recovery in mental illness. The immune system seems to play what was, until recently, an underappreciated role in brain and mind function. Therapies based on drugs that act through the immune system are in trials and causing excitement while, at the same time, the immune system may be involved, in part, in the mechanisms of some talking or contemplative therapies. Related to this, the role of the millions of gut bacteria we live with, the microbiota, is also causing a stir in mental and physical health. Both the immune system and the gut microbiota may hold part of the answer as to why mental illness is so often associated with physical ill health[1,2] and why, beyond the terrible sadness of deaths from suicide, people with mental illness die too soon from a host of physical illnesses.[3] It is vital that we get over the mental–physical divide, not least for health services and research funders.

Readers may have noticed the similarities between different mental health disorders. Just as mental health sciences involve intersections, people with lived experience and clinicians, families, carers and supporters know that there are many overlaps between these conditions, at any one time and over time. Similarly, there is a great deal of overlap in the factors we consider as contributing to causes of mental ill health, including genetic factors and harmful environmental factors such as adverse events in childhood. This is reflected in a new way of thinking known as transdiagnostic, where traditional diagnostic boundaries are blurred. I am confident that such transdiagnostic thinking will bring great dividends, not least as mental health researchers realise that their findings may have a great deal to say about conditions that they believed were in the realm of others. Together with crossing the mind–brain–body divide, this kind of transdiagnostic thinking is exciting in the potential it holds.

Perhaps the boldest, most creative example of transdiagnostic thinking in the book is Chapter 5 on self-destructive behaviour. Few will be familiar with the juxtaposition of suicide and deliberate self-harm (also known as non-suicidal self-injury, among other terms) with addictions and harmful gambling. But some of the mechanisms of these seemingly disparate conditions, such as ruminations and abnormal reward pathways, may be common to them all. This arrangement is not intended to make readers uncomfortable, but to help them see serious problems in a new light, offering cross-diagnostic strategies.

The book focuses particularly but not exclusively on disorders that have depression and anxiety at their core. A number of conditions are absent and these include schizophrenia and other psychotic disorders, such as bipolar disorder, or personality disorders (PD).

It is these disorders that were more in the realm of the mental asylums that Bill Bryson refers to in his introduction, in which he recalls working during the 1970s at Holloway Sanatorium, to the north-west of London. There wasn't a great deal of mental health science supporting asylum practice during the nineteenth century and first half of the twentieth century; rather it was fuelled by moral virtue and the values of the time; though, as Bryson points out, there were efforts to be kind and therapeutic, even if they now look hopelessly misplaced.

That said, observational research 100 years ago by those such as Alzheimer, Kraepelin and the Bleulers (father and son) still influences ideas about mental health diagnosis today. Many people who spent years in asylums lived with what we might today see as schizophrenia, bipolar disorder or long-term, severe depression (in the past called melancholia), overlaid by the effects of institutionalisation and a range of organic brain diseases such as syphilis, or conditions like nutritional deficiencies.

In the UK, the asylums began to empty over the middle five decades of the century. One of the first was Mapperley Hospital on the outskirts of Nottingham, where the physician-superintendent in the 1940s was Dr Duncan Macmillan. He questioned whether his long-term patients really should be removed from society. He opened the gates and found patients and the local community did perfectly well, and community care was born – nearly a decade before the advent of antipsychotic drugs such as chlorpromazine. Macmillan wrote to the medical journal the *Lancet*, and hospitals gradually followed his lead, no doubt supported by the new pharmacological agents.

As people were discharged from mental asylums it was assumed that those who went to live with their families would fare better than those who went to lodging houses. On the contrary, it was those who spent a great deal of time with their families who were more likely to relapse and have to return to hospital. The key to this effect was linked to high emotional tone in families, consisting of critical comments, over-involvement and hostility, sometimes tempered by positive comments and warmth.

Through education about the mental health condition of their relative, along with reducing face-to-face contact, this expressed emotion in families could be lowered and relapses avoided. Clinical trials were done, the approach codified as 'family intervention' delivered by trained practitioners, and it is now an accepted part of clinical practice, and woven into other therapeutic modalities.

It's a fascinating story[4] and sets the scene for an important principle of twenty-first-century mental healthcare: the triangle of care where planning and delivery of interventions and care are based on mutually respectful conversations and understanding between the person with lived experience, the carer(s) and mental health and care professionals. My reason for setting out this piece of history is to suggest that conversations about cutting-edge research ought to involve a similar range of voices from lived experience, carers, healthcare professionals and researchers – perhaps the care diamond or four-square of care.

To be fair, mental health research is more advanced than other areas of health research in engaging, including and involving people with lived experience of mental ill health and the general population in its research. This now has a theoretical framework, and virtually always results in better research and faster implementation, but it's very rare to have the kind of high-quality, unplugged candour in those conversations, from both sides, that we can construct from these pages. We just need to make the exchanges real.

That being said, the potential audiences for this book are obvious: anyone interested in or who experiences mental illnesses, those who provide care, their families, mental health scientists and those who fund them. They, too, are stakeholders in the interdisciplinary approach the book supports. I would particularly recommend the book to non-clinical researchers at all stages of their careers. Everyone needs to get involved in conversations and share ideas about mental health science research.

After all, without research, it's just guesswork.

Declaration of interest: Professor Jones is a charity trustee and chair of Mental Health Science Council at MQ: Mental Health Research, and a charity trustee at Mental Health Research UK. He is also honorary consultant psychiatrist at the Cambridgeshire and Peterborough NHS Foundation Trust.

endnotes

FOREWORD

1 Billy Monger interviewed by Ed Jackson, 'It's Good to Walk' [podcast], 2021, https://podcasts.apple.com/us/podcast/7-the-power-of-positivity-billy-monger/id1555214234?i=1000517704330

2 Bryson, Bill, *Notes From a Small Island*, (Doubleday, 1995)

3 Gawande, Atul, *The Checklist Manifesto: How to Get Things Right*, (Metropolitan Books, 2009)

INTRODUCTION

1 https://www.lse.ac.uk/News/Latest-news-from-LSE/2022/c-Mar-22/Mental-health-problems-cost-UK-economy-at-least-118-billion-a-year-new-research#:~:text=Mental%20health%20problems%20cost%20the,cent%20of%20the%20UK's%20GDP

2 https://www.mqmentalhealth.org/wp-content/uploads/UKMentalHealthResearchFunding2014-2017digital.pdf

DEPRESSION

1 Source: Prof. Brenda Pennix, Amsterdam,

2 https://www.sciencedirect.com/science/article/pii/S0022395621002211?via%3Dihub

3 Flouri, E et al. 'Prenatal and childhood adverse life events, inflammation and depressive symptoms across adolescence' *Journal of Affective Disorders*, Vol. 260: 577–582. https://www.sciencedirect.com/science/article/pii/S0165032719314296?via%3Dihub

4 https://www.nature.com/articles/mp201567

5   https://www.mqmentalhealth.org/research/identifying-depression-early-in-adolescence-idea/

6   Barnett K, Mercer SW, Norbury M, Watt G, Wyke S, Guthrie B. (2012). 'Epidemiology of multimorbidity and implications for health care, research, and medical education: a crosssectional study'. *The Lancet* online

7   Benros ME, Waltoft BL, Nordentoft M et al. 'Autoimmune diseases and severe infections as risk factors for mood disorders: a nationwide study'. *JAMA Psychiatry*. 2013;70(8):812–20 https:// jamanetwork.com/journals/jamapsychiatry/fullarticle/ 1696348

8   Zheng Y et al. 'Role of Inflammation in Depression and Anxiety: Tests for Disorder Specificity, Linearity and Potential Causality of Association'. UK Biobank. https://www.medrxiv.org/content/ 10.1101/2021.02.02.21250987v1

9   Pitharouli MC et al. 'Elevated C-Reactive Protein in Patients With Depression, Independent of Genetic, Health, and Psychosocial Factors: Results From the UK Biobank'. *American Journal of Psychiatry*, Vol. 179, No. 1

10 Strawbridge R et al. 'Inflammatory profiles of severe treatment-resistant depression'. *Journal of Affective Disorders*, Vol. 146: 42–51. https://www.sciencedirect.com/science/article/pii/ S0165032718318561?via%3Dihub

11 Kim SJ et al. 'Cd4+cd25+ regulatory t cell depletion modulates anxiety and depression-like behaviors in mice'. *PLoS One*, 7 (2012), 10.1371/journal.pone.0042054

12 Pace TW et al. 'Increased stress-induced inflammatory responses in male patients with major depression and increased early life stress'. *Am J Psychiatry*. 2006;163:1630-1633. https://ajp.psychiatryonline. org/doi/full/10.1176/ajp.2006.163.9.1630

13 Nettis, Maria Antionetta et al. 'Augmentation therapy with minocycline in treatment-resistant depression patients with low-grade peripheral inflammation: results from a double-blind randomised clinical trial'. *Journal of Neuropsychopharmacology*. doi: 10.1038/s41386-020-00948-6. Epub 2021 Jan 28.

14 https://www.nhlbi.nih.gov/news/2017/heart-disease-and-depression-two-way-relationship

15 'Shared mechanisms between coronary heart disease and depression. Findings from a large UK general population-based cohort'. *Molecular Psychiatry*. https://www.sciencedirect.com/science/article/pii/S0306453020301013?via%3Dihub

16 Avon Longitudinal Study of Parents and Children | Avon Longitudinal Study of Parents and Children | University of Bristol

17 'Cardiometabolic risk in young adults with depression and evidence of inflammation. A birth cohort study'. *Psychoneuroendocrinology*. https://www.sciencedirect.com/science/article/pii/S0306453020301013?via%3Dihub

18 Andersson et al. 'Depression and the risk of autoimmune disease: a nationally representative, prospective longitudinal study'. *Psychological Medicine* (2015), 45, 3559–3569. Cambridge University Press 2015 doi:10.1017/S0033291715001488.

19 Tubbs JD et al. 'Immune dysregulation in depression. Evidence from genome-wide association'. *Brain, Behaviour & Immunity*, Vol. 7. https://www.sciencedirect.com/science/article/pii/S2666354620300739

20 Maxwell J et al. 'Association Between Genetic Risk for Psychiatric Disorders and the Probability of Living in Urban Settings'. *JAMA Psychiatry*. https://jamanetwork.com/journals/jamapsychiatry/article-abstract/2785027

21 Mackes NK et al. 'Early childhood deprivation is associated with alterations in adult brain structure despite subsequent environmental enrichment'. Proceedings of the National Academy of Sciences. 117 (1) 641–649. https://www.pnas.org/doi/full/10.1073/pnas.1911264116

22 https://www.spectrumnews.org/news/autistic-burnout-explained/

23 https://polaristeen.com/articles/how-many-teens-have-depression/

24 https://www.psychiatrictimes.com/view/bereavement-related-depression

25 https://pubmed.ncbi.nlm.nih.gov/2185504/

26 https://journals.co.za/doi/abs/10.10520/EJC108933

27 https://www.sciencedirect.com/science/article/pii/
S0885392401003633.

28 https://www.sciencedirect.com/science/article/abs/pii/
S0165032714004972?via%3Dihub

29 Goldie Sayers, a GB Olympic medallist in the javelin carried out
significant research on this topic during her Masters studies at
Salford University. Her advice on this section was extremely
valuable. Dissertation is available from the University.

30 https://onlinelibrary.wiley.com/doi/full/10.1002/jclp.23192

31 https://pubmed.ncbi.nlm.nih.gov/29508381/

32 https://onlinelibrary.wiley.com/doi/epdf/10.1002/ijop.12483

ANXIETY

1 Lee WE, Wadsworth MEJ, Hotopf A. The protective role of trait anxiety:
A longitudinal cohort study. Psychol Med. 2006;36(3):345–351.
https://www.cambridge.org/core/journals/psychological-medicine/
article/abs/protective-role-of-trait-anxiety-a-longitudinal-cohort-
study/919A2F6F0C52E512A5F67E3AFE7B7A0F

2 Mykletun A, Bjerkeset O, Overland S. Levels of anxiety and depression
as predictors of mortality: The HUNT study. Br J Psychiatry.
2009;195(2):118–125. https://www.cambridge.org/core/journals/
the-british-journal-of-psychiatry/article/levels-of-anxiety-and-
depression-aspredictors-of-mortality-the-hunt-study/
E5415752846D3F6C5408BEB06016A9E7

3 Tali Manber Ball, Sarah Sullivan, Taru Flagan, Carla A Hitchcock, Alan
Simmons, Martin P Paulus, Murray B Stein, Selective eff ects of social
anxiety, anxiety sensitivity, and negative aff ectivity on the neural
bases of emotional face processing. NeuroImage, Vol. 59, Issue 2,
Pages 1879–1887, https://doi.org/10.1016/j.neuroimage.2011.08.074

4 Ochsner KN, Silvers JA, Buhle JT. Functional imaging studies of
emotion regulation: a synthetic review and evolving model of the
cognitive control of emotion. Ann N Y Acad Sci. 2012;1251:E1–E24.
doi:10.1111/j.1749-6632.2012.06751.x

5 Reinoud Kaldewaij, Andrea Reinecke, Catherine J Harmer. A lack of differentiation in amygdala responses to fearful expression intensity in panic disorder patients. Psychiatry Research: Neuroimaging, Vol. 291, Pages 18–25. https://doi.org/10.1016/j.pscychresns.2019.07.002

6 https://www.nature.com/articles/s41398-018-0277-5

7 https://med.stanford.edu/news/all-news/2009/12/brain-scans-show-distinctive-patterns-inpeople-with-generalized-anxiety-disorder-in-stanford-study.html

8 https://www.medicalnewstoday.com/articles/anxiety-disorder-abnormal-heart-brain-connectionidentified#Surprising-results

9 Colette R Hirsch, Andrew Mathews. A cognitive model of pathological worry. Behaviour Research and Therapy, Vol. 50, Issue 10, Pages 636–646. https://doi.org/10.1016/j.brat.2012.06.007

10 Claire Eagleson, Sarra Hayes, Andrew Mathews, Gemma Perman, Colette R Hirsch. The power of positive thinking: Pathological worry is reduced by thought replacement in Generalized Anxiety Disorder. Behaviour Research and Therapy, Vol. 78, Pages 13–18. https://doi.org/10.1016/j.brat.2015.12.01

11 Hirsch CR, Krahé C, Whyte J, Bridge L, Loizou S, Norton S, Mathews A. (2020). Effects of modifying interpretation bias on transdiagnostic repetitive negative thinking. Journal of Consulting and Clinical Psychology, 88(3), 226–239. https://doi.org/10.1037/ccp0000455

12 https://www.sciencedirect.com/science/article/abs/pii/S000579671400120X?via%3Dihub

13 Andrea Reinecke, Alecia Nickless, Michael Browning, Catherine J Harmer. Neurocognitive processes in d-cycloserine augmented single-session exposure therapy for anxiety: A randomized placebo-controlled trial. Behaviour Research and Therapy, Vol. 129. https://doi.org/10.1016/j.brat.2020.103607

14 Graham BM, Milad MR. (2013). Blockade of Estrogen by Hormonal Contraceptives Impairs Fear Extinction in Female Rats and Women. Biological Psychiatry 73(4); DOI:10.1016/j.biopsych.2012.09.018;

15 Graham BM, Milad MR. (2014). Inhibition of estradiol synthesis impairs fear extinction in male rats. PMID: 24939838, PMCID: PMC4061425, DOI: 10.1101/lm.034926.114

16 Op cit, Graham and Gilad 2013

17 Graham et al. (2018). The association between estradiol levels, hormonal contraceptive use, and responsiveness to one-session-treatment for spider phobia in women. Psychoneuroendocrinology, Vol. 90, April 2018, Pages 134–140

18 Graham BM, Milad MR. (2013). Blockade of Estrogen by Hormonal Contraceptives Impairs Fear Extinction in Female Rats and Women. Biological Psychiatry 73(4); DOI:10.1016/j.biopsych.2012.09.018;

19 https://acamh.onlinelibrary.wiley.com/doi/full/10.1111/jcpp.12809?casa_token=QMjKi6BnwqIAAAAA%3AUDe-hTgUV_Wgd-c7unsbiMEZDONqMJg0XxeVpffE2iUa9AYawcy-ob30s7QCy7FoC0aTVgB0AcAqjof1

20 Kacper Łoś, Napoleon Waszkiewicz. Biological Markers in Anxiety Disorders. Journal of Clinical Medicine, Vol. 10, Issue 8, 10.3390/jcm10081744

21 John A et al. (2021). Association of school absence and exclusion with recorded neurodevelopmental disorders, mental disorders, or self-harm: a nationwide, retrospective, electronic cohort study of children and young people in Wales, UK. Lancet (Psychiatry) Vol. 9 (1) pp 23–34, January 2022

PTSD

1 https://www.cambridge.org/core/journals/psychological-medicine/article/intrusive-memories-to-traumatic-footage-the-neural-basis-of-their-encoding-and-involuntary-recall/4ECBEF5098CBA-21F95A9C546D5CBE54E

2 https://www.ncbi.nlm.nih.gov/pmc/articles/PMC6760386/pdf/arh-23-4-256.pdf

3 https://www.alcoholrehabguide.org/resources/dual-diagnosis/alcohol-and-ptsd

4 https://drugfree.org/drug-and-alcohol-news/high-rates-of-childhood-trauma-found-in-adult-alcoholics

5 https://jamanetwork.com/journals/jamapsychiatry/fullarticle/210821

6 https://www.tandfonline.com/doi/abs/10.1080/15289168.2011.575704

7 https://www.cambridge.org/core/journals/psychological-medicine/article/prospective-study-of-pretrauma-risk-factors-for-posttraumatic-stress-disorder-and-depression/AD48BA08F79F2D3D3CF1A10BEECD2B6C

8 https://bmjopen.bmj.com/content/8/12/bmjopen-2018-022292

9 https://journals.sagepub.com/doi/pdf/10.1177/1099800418800396

10 https://bpspsychub.onlinelibrary.wiley.com/doi/10.1111/bjc.12340

11 https://www.mqmentalhealth.org/new-ptsd-treatment

12 Horsch, A. et al. (2017) 'Reducing intrusive traumatic memories after emergency caesarean section: a proof-of-principle randomized controlled study.' *Behav. Res. Ther.* 94, 36–47

13 Iyadurai, L. et al. 'Preventing intrusive memories after trauma via a brief intervention involving Tetris computer game play in the emergency department: a proof-of-concept randomized controlled trial.' *Mol. Psychiatry* 23, 28 March 2017, 674–682 (2018)

14 Kessler, H. et al. 'Reducing intrusive memories of trauma using a visuospatial interference intervention with inpatients with posttraumatic stress disorder (PTSD).' *J. Consult. Clin. Psychol.* 86, 1076–1090 (2018)

15 https://adc.bmj.com/content/105/4/347

16 https://bmcmedicine.biomedcentral.com/articles/10.1186/s12916-022-02329-w

17 https://www.thelancet.com/journals/lanpsy/article/PIIS2215-0366(21)00367-9/fulltext

EATING DISORDERS

1 https://www.beateatingdisorders.org.uk/about-beat/policy-work/policy-and-best-practice-reports/prevalence-in-the-uk

2 https://www.england.nhs.uk/statistics/statistical-work-areas/cyped-waiting-times

3 The Cost of Eating Disorders in the UK 2019 and 2020, Hearts Minds and Genes Coalition. (2021). https://www.pslhub.org/learn/patient-safety-in-health-and-care/mental-health/eating-disorders/the-cost-of-eating-disorders-in-the-uk-2019-and-2020-24-september-2021-r5242/

4 https://pubmed.ncbi.nlm.nih.gov/28680630/

5 https://www.frontiersin.org/articles/10.3389/fnins.2019.00596/full

6 https://www.frontiersin.org/articles/10.3389/fpsyg.2019.02200/full

7 https://edgiuk.org/

8 https://www.biologicalpsychiatryjournal.com/article/S0006-3223(22)01290-2/fulltext

9 https://go.gale.com/ps/i.do?id=GALE%7CA366729907&sid=googleScholar&v=2.1&it=r&linkaccess=abs&issn=08932905&p=AONE&sw=w&userGroupName=anon%7E359ef2b8

10 https://jamanetwork.com/journals/jamapsychiatry/fullarticle/1108406

11 https://journals.plos.org/plosone/article?id=10.1371/journal.pone.0022259

12 https://www.ncbi.nlm.nih.gov/pmc/articles/PMC4543093/

13 https://jamanetwork.com/journals/jamapsychiatry/fullarticle/2781384

14 https://www.biologicalpsychiatryjournal.com/article/S0006-3223(20)31672-3/fulltext

15 https://jeatdisord.biomedcentral.com/articles/10.1186/s40337-020-00312-5

16 https://www.frontiersin.org/articles/10.3389/fpsyt.2019.00635/full#B2

17 https://www.sciencedirect.com/science/article/pii/S2352250X21000397#bib33

18 https://jeatdisord.biomedcentral.com/articles/10.1186/s40337-021-00424-6

19 https://onlinelibrary.wiley.com/doi/full/10.1002/eat.23556

20 https://pubmed.ncbi.nlm.nih.gov/24888426/

21 https://akjournals.com/view/journals/2006/5/1/article-p11.xml

22 https://www.sciencedirect.com/science/article/pii/
S0195666312002243

23 https://academic.oup.com/ajcn/article/94/6/1562/4598194

24 https://www.sciencedirect.com/science/article/abs/pii/
S0031938415300226

25 https://www.mqmentalhealth.org/research/understanding-the-
role-of-appetite-in-thedevelopment-of-eating-disorders/

26 https://academic.oup.com/ajcn/article/103/1/231/4662861

27 https://freedfromed.co.uk/

28 https://www.nature.com/articles/s41398-020-00977-1

29 https://clinicaltrials.gov/ct2/show/NCT04778423

30 https://bmjopen.bmj.com/content/bmjopen/8/7/e021531.full.pdf

31 https://jeatdisord.biomedcentral.com/articles/10.1186/s40337-021-
00420-w

32 https://onlinelibrary.wiley.com/doi/10.1002/eat.23267

33 https://www.ncbi.nlm.nih.gov/pmc/articles/PMC3961475/?tool=nihms

34 Kalfoglou Andrea. (2016). Ethical and Clinical Dilemmas in Using
Psychotropic Medications During Pregnancy. AMA Journal of ethics.
18. 614–623. 10.1001/journalofethics.2016.18.6.stas1–1606

35 Hippman C, Balneaves LG. Women's decision making about
antidepressant use during pregnancy: A narrative review, 2018.
https://doi.org/10.1002/da.22821

36 https://onlinelibrary.wiley.com/doi/full/10.1002/jgc4.1049

SELF-DESTRUCTIVE BEHAVIOURS

1 https://openaccess.city.ac.uk/id/eprint/23646/

2 https://www.mentalhealth.org.uk/explore-mental-health/statistics/
men-women-statistics

3 https://adc.bmj.com/content/105/4/347#ref-10

4 https://adc.bmj.com/content/105/4/347.info

5 https://emj.bmj.com/content/37/12/752

6 https://www.sciencedirect.com/science/article/pii/S0165032716
303585

7 https://www.sciencedirect.com/science/article/pii/S016503272
0328706?via%3Dihub

8 https://www.cambridge.org/core/journals/the-british-journal-of-
psychiatry/article/impact-of-thecovid19-pandemic-on-presentations-
to-health-services-following-selfh arm-systematic-review/
DE39F96D7FD96F88508C6097398E806D

9 https://bmcmedicine.biomedcentral.com/articles/10.1186/s12916-
022-02329-w

10 https://bmcpsychiatry.biomedcentral.com/articles/10.1186/s12888-
019-2350-x

11 https://journals.sagepub.com/doi/full/10.1177/1461444819850106

12 https://journals.lww.com/indianjpsychiatry/Fulltext/2018/60040/
The_role_of_online_social_networking_on_deliberate.3.aspx

13 https://3syp.com/

14 https://www.ncbi.nlm.nih.gov/pmc/articles/PMC3164585/

15 https://www.tandfonline.com/doi/abs/10.1080/14659890500114359

16 https://link.springer.com/book/10.1007/978-3-031-04772-5

17 https://www.frontiersin.org/articles/10.3389/fpsyt.2018.00166/full

18 Ashton, H. & Golding, J. (1989). Smoking and Human Behaviour.
Chichester: John Wiley & Sons Inc.

19 Griffiths, M.D. & Calado, F. (2022). Gambling disorder. In Pontes, H.
(Ed.), Behavioral Addictions: Conceptual, Clinical, Assessment, and
Treatment Approaches (pp.1–29). Cham: Springer.

20 https://www.mdpi.com/2075-4426/12/5/690

21 https://onlinelibrary.wiley.com/doi/abs/10.1046/j.1360-
0443.1999.9479814.x

22 https://onlinelibrary.wiley.com/doi/abs/10.1046/j.1360-0443.2000.9568735.x

23 Griffiths, M.D. & Calado, F. (2022). Gambling disorder. In Pontes, H. (Ed.), Behavioral Addictions: Conceptual, Clinical, Assessment, and Treatment Approaches (pp.1–29). Cham: Springer.

24 Ibid.

25 Orford, J. (2001). Excessive Appetites: A Psychological View of the Addictions (Second Edition). Chichester: Wiley

26 https://ajph.aphapublications.org/doi/abs/10.2105/AJPH.84.2.237

27 https://cdspress.ca/wp-content/uploads/2022/07/Rachel-A.-Volberg-1-1.pdf

28 https://bpspsychub.onlinelibrary.wiley.com/doi/10.1111/j.2044-8295.1994.tb02529.x

29 https://psycnet.apa.org/record/1976-07038-001

30 McMurran, M. (1994). The Psychology of Addiction. London: Taylor and Francis.

31 https://juniperpublishers.com/gjarm/pdf/GJARM.MS.ID.555610.pdf

32 https://psycnet.apa.org/doiLanding?doi=10.1037%2F0022-006X.56.2.183

33 https://www.kcl.ac.uk/research/sure-substance-use-recovery-evaluator

34 https://bpspsychub.onlinelibrary.wiley.com/doi/10.1111/j.2044-8295.1994.tb02529.x

35 http://www.meta-systems.eu/nickbrown/blog/griffiths/exhibit3/sp103%20(Annotated)%20Griffiths%20-%202011%20-%20Adolescent%20Gambling.pdf

36 Ibid.

37 https://bpspsychub.onlinelibrary.wiley.com/doi/10.1348/0007 12699161503

38 https://www.academia.edu/780647/Griffiths_M.D._and_Parke_J._2003_._The_environmental_psychology_of_gambling._In_G._Reith_

Ed._Gambling_Who_wins_Who_Loses_pp._277-292._New_York_
Prometheus_Books

39 https://www.frontiersin.org/articles/10.3389/fpsyg.2012.00621/full

40 https://onlinelibrary.wiley.com/doi/abs/10.1111/sltb.12450

41 https://journals.sagepub.com/doi/10.1177/1403494817746274

42 https://www.ncbi.nlm.nih.gov/pmc/articles/PMC7955273/

43 https://ajp.psychiatryonline.org/doi/10.1176/appi.ajp.2016.16010077

44 https://jamanetwork.com/journals/jamanetworkopen/fullarticle/
2788456

45 https://bmjopen.bmj.com/content/11/12/e053808

46 https://www.ncbi.nlm.nih.gov/pmc/articles/PMC8136175

47 https://www.sciencedirect.com/science/article/abs/pii/
S0140673612603225

48 https://www.sciencedirect.com/science/article/pii/S22150366
19300306

49 https://suicidalbehaviourresearchlab.files.wordpress.com/2022/
07/1-s2.0-s0277953622001666-main.pdf

50 https://suicidalbehaviourresearchlab.files.wordpress.com/2022/07/
autism_and_autistic_traits_in_those_who_died_by_suicide_in_
england.pdf

51 https://www.sciencedirect.com/science/article/abs/pii/
S0165032719329726

52 https://suicidalbehaviourresearchlab.files.wordpress.com/2022/07/
psychosocial-factors-thatdistinguish-between-men-and-women-who-
have-suicidal-thoughts-and-attempt-suicidefindings-from-a-national-
probability-sample-of-adults-div.pdf

53 https://www.sciencedirect.com/science/article/pii/S016517
8119315938

54 https://www.sciencedirect.com/science/article/abs/pii/
S0022395621004398?via%3Dihub

55 https://www.sciencedirect.com/science/article/abs/pii/S00223956
19303115?via%3Dihub

56 https://www.sciencedirect.com/science/article/abs/pii/S016503
2718312898?via%3Dihub

57 https://www.sciencedirect.com/science/article/abs/pii/S030645
3016308435

58 https://suicidalbehaviourresearchlab.files.wordpress.com/2022/
07/1-s2.0-s0022395621005057-main.pdf

59 https://bmcpsychiatry.biomedcentral.com/articles/10.1186/s12888-
018-1910-9

60 https://www.sciencedirect.com/science/article/abs/pii/
S0890856709601659

61 https://static.homepagetool.ch/var/m_6/60/605/202013/9563828-
PLOS_Medicine_2016_03_02.PDF

62 https://static.homepagetool.ch/var/m_6/60/605/202013/9563822-
JAMA_Network_2018_10_18.pdf

63 https://cams-care.com/about-cams/

64 https://www.frontiersin.org/articles/10.3389/fpsyt.2018.00567/full

65 https://akjournals.com/view/journals/2006/11/1/article-p128.xml

66 https://www.dovepress.com/articles.php?article_id=72260

67 https://www.begambleaware.org/sites/default/files/2020-12/
suicide-report_0.pdf

68 https://www.sciencedirect.com/science/article/pii/S221503
6619300306

69 https://www.nature.com/articles/s41598-018-25773-2

70 https://journals.plos.org/plosone/article?id=10.1371/journal.
pone.0253809

71 https://link.springer.com/article/10.1007/s11469-020-00462-2

72 https://bmcpsychiatry.biomedcentral.com/articles/10.1186/s12888-
021-03268-1

73 https://akjournals.com/view/journals/2006/11/1/article-p128.xml

74 https://www.frontiersin.org/articles/10.3389/fpsyt.2017.00027/
full#B18

SPOTLIGHT ON AGEING HAPPILY

1 https://onlinelibrary.wiley.com/doi/10.1002/cne.901240303

2 https://www.cell.com/fulltext/S0092-8674(13)00533-3

3 https://www.science.org/doi/10.1126/science.1173215

4 https://www.frontiersin.org/articles/10.3389/fnins.2017.00571/full

5 https://onlinelibrary.wiley.com/doi/10.1111/j.1474-9726.2006.00197.x

6 https://www.sciencedirect.com/science/article/pii/S0006295217
304392#b0140

7 https://www.sciencedirect.com/science/article/abs/pii/S09594
38814001743?via%3Dihub

8 https://physoc.onlinelibrary.wiley.com/doi/full/10.1113/JP271270

9 https://www.jneurosci.org/content/25/38/8680

10 https://www.sciencedirect.com/science/article/pii/S108707920
8000804?via%3Dihub

11 https://www.nature.com/articles/s41380-021-01102-4

12 Lee J, Seroogy KB, Mattson MP (2002) Dietary restriction enhances
neurotrophin expression and neurogenesis in the hippocampus of
adult mice. J Neurochem 80:539–547

13 Aoki H, Kimoto K, Hori N, Toyoda M (2005) Cell proliferation in the
dentate gyrus of rat hippocampus is inhibited by soft diet feeding.
Gerontology 51:369–374

14 https://www.mdpi.com/2072-6643/13/6/2067

15 https://www.tandfonline.com/doi/full/10.31887/DCNS.2019.21.1/
nscarmeas

16 Ng TP, Chiam PC, Lee T, Chua HC, Lim L, Kua EH (2006) Curry
consumption and cognitive function in the elderly. Am J Epidemiol
164:898–906

17 https://www.nature.com/articles/s42003-020-0844-1

18 https://www.nature.com/articles/s41380-022-01644-1

19 https://pubmed.ncbi.nlm.nih.gov/28033521/

20 https://www.sciencedirect.com/science/article/pii/
S0149763419305640

21 https://onlinelibrary.wiley.com/doi/full/10.1002/da.22915?casa_
token=JOn2sFeezvkAAAAA%3AuN-LXc4X-5AYVbuhRrsqNkrpm2QqGB
bxMxd91W-iHzcWLUgHzLRzUthkrd8yTH27o2bbw5BsRhHHHd4&sa
ml_referrer

22 https://academic.oup.com/nutritionreviews/article/76/7/481/4985
887?login=false

23 https://ieeexplore.ieee.org/abstract/document/8110878?casa_toke
n=jPF6rjT9M44AAAAA:jCPqxINikzYndsAY2raxPMcG0kFYOa68_
VeWW_oi3L3IGJqpbRei2dCw6ttrk26QRqHEj_M

24 https://www.ncbi.nlm.nih.gov/pmc/articles/PMC7510518/

25 https://www.sciencedirect.com/science/article/pii/S088915911
5000884?via%3Dihub

26 https://www.nature.com/articles/s41467-022-34502-3

27 https://alz-journals.onlinelibrary.wiley.com/doi/full/10.1002/
alz.12428

CONCLUSION

1 Momen, N.C., Plana-Ripoll, O., Agerbo, E., Benros, M.E. et al. (2020)
'Association between Mental Disorders and Subsequent Medical
Conditions'. *N Engl J Med.* Apr 30;382(18):1721–1731. doi:10.1056/
NEJMoa1915784

2 Plana-Ripoll, O., Pedersen, C.B., Holtz, Y., Benros, M.E. et al. (2019)
'Exploring Comorbidity Within Mental Disorders Among a Danish
National Population.' *JAMA Psychiatry.* Mar 1;76(3):259–270.
doi:10.1001/jamapsychiatry.2018.3658

3 Momen, N.C., Plana-Ripoll, O., Agerbo, E., Christensen, M.K. et al.
(2022) 'Mortality Associated With Mental Disorders and Comorbid

General Medical Conditions.' *JAMA Psychiatry*. May 1;79(5):444–453. doi:10.1001/jamapsychiatry.2022.0347

4 Peter B. Jones and S. Marder (2008) 'Psychosocial and pharmacological treatments for schizophrenia.' In: Tyrer and Silk (eds.), *Cambridge Textbook of Effective Treatments in Psychiatry*. doi:10.1017/CBO9780511544392.028

acknowledgements

Thank you to Peter George and Andy Leaver for their unwavering support for this project, as well as all of those who have contributed to this book by telling their most personal stories.

index

Note: page numbers in **bold** refer to diagrams, page numbers in *italics* refer to information contained in tables.